£1·00

HOMEOPATHY

PETER ADAMS is a Registered Homeopath and joint owner of Stroud Natural Health Clinic in Gloucestershire, where twelve alternative/complementary medical systems are provided.

D0532346

THE SERIES

New Perspectives provide attractive and accessible introductions to a comprehensive range of mind, body and spirit topics. Beautifully designed and illustrated, these practical books are written by experts in each subject.

Titles in the series include:

ALEXANDER TECHNIQUE
by Richard Brennan

MASSAGE
by Stewart Mitchell

AROMATHERAPY
by Christine Wildwood

MEDITATION
by David Fontana

DREAMS
by David Fontana

NLP
by Carol Harris

FENG SHUI
by Man-Ho Kwok with Joanne O'Brien

NUMEROLOGY
by Rodford Barrat

FLOWER REMEDIES
by Christine Wildwood

REFLEXOLOGY
by Inge Dougans

HOMEOPATHY
by Peter Adams

TAROT
by A T Mann

New Perspectives

HOMEOPATHY

An Introductory Guide to Natural Medicine for the Whole Person

PETER ADAMS

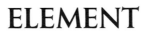

ELEMENT

Shaftesbury, Dorset • Boston, Massachusetts
Melbourne, Victoria

First published as *Health Essentials: Homeopathy*
in 1996 by Element Books Limited

This revised edition first published in Great Britain in 1999 by
Element Books Limited, Shaftesbury, Dorset SP7 8BP

Published in the USA in 1999 by Element Books, Inc.
160 North Washington Street, Boston, MA 02114

Published in Australia in 1999 by
Element Books and distributed by
Penguin Australia Limited
487 Maroondah Highway,
Ringwood, Victoria 3134

Designed for Element Books Limited by
Design Revolution, Queens Park Villa,
30 West Drive, Brighton, East Sussex BN2 2GE

ELEMENT BOOKS LIMITED
Editorial Director: Sarah Sutton
Editorial Manager: Jane Pizzey
Commissioning Editor: Grace Cheetham
Production Director: Roger Lane

DESIGN REVOLUTION
Editorial Director: Ian Whitelaw
Art Director: Lindsey Johns
Editor: Julie Whitaker
Designer: Vanessa Good

Printed and bound in Great Britain by
Bemrose Security Printing, Derby

British Library Cataloguing in Publication
data available

Library of Congress Cataloging in Publication
data available

ISBN 1-86204-663-8

CONTENTS

Acknowledgements and Dedication

I would like to thank everyone who helped with this book. My patients who allowed me to us their case notes; friends and family who commented on the manuscript; homeopaths Julian Carlyon, Rissa Carlyon, Simon Eiles and Joy Adams; Anja Liengaard who introduced me to homeopathy; Paul Jackson of Original Business Systems; Julia McCutchen at Element Books for giving me the opportunity to write. Finally I thank my family for giving me the time, and my parents for being my parents. This book is dedicated to them, Margaret and Ralph.

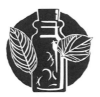

INTRODUCTION

Homeopathy is definitely a growth area and becomes more popular every year. A steady stream of television and radio programmes and regular newspaper and magazine articles have appeared in response to increased interest in this system of complementary medicine.

Sales of homeopathic medicines are increasing every year, and doubled in Britain between 1989 and 1994. A leading national pharmacy chain is now marketing its own brand in Britain. Homeopathy is definitely a growth area. In Europe during the 1980s its rate of growth was second only to the computer industry.

Private health insurance schemes now often include the option of homeopathic treatment in their policies in response to an increased demand from the public for professional homeopathic treatment for more serious problems.

Orthodox medical interest is growing, too. Articles on homeopathy now appear more frequently in scientific and medical journals. More trials are being conducted showing the effectiveness of homeopathic remedies. A survey of trials of homeopathy published in the *British Medical Journal* in February 1991 concluded:

> *'The amount of positive evidence...*
> *came as a surprise to us. Based on this evidence*
> *we would be ready to accept that homeopathy*
> *can be efficacious, if only the mechanism of action*
> *were more plausible.'*

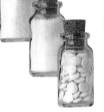

LEFT HOMEOPATHIC REMEDIES ARE EXTREMELY EASY TO USE, WHICH MAKES THEM VERY POPULAR IN THE HOME FOR FIRST AID AND FOR COMMON ILLNESSES.

I understand the scepticism of the medical establishment very well because I subscribed to it myself until 20 years ago. However I was forced by the facts to change my mind.

I lived on a smallholding and had a cow that had a dislocated knee cap. The veterinary surgeon could do nothing and there was a possibility that the animal would require an operation. A friend, to whom I will always be grateful, heard of my plight. She appeared with a little brown envelope containing some small round pills, together with instructions on how to administer them to the cow. Those pills and those strange instructions will be familiar to many of you, but to me at that time they were an amusing eccentricity. I followed the instructions, and went to bed that night without thinking any more of it.

The following day I went to the cow's open shed but she wasn't there. I looked out and saw her ambling slowly and peacefully across the field, grazing with that timeless pace cows have. She needed a repeat dose of the remedy a few days later and another one after the next calving, but apart from that the problem never returned. (The remedy, by the way, was *rhus tox*.)

Although still unconvinced by homeopathic theory I was now intrigued. This seemed like magic. How did these little pills with hardly anything in them cure my cow, a beast totally immune to the placebo effect?

LEFT THE REMEDY *RHUS TOX.*, WHICH IS MADE FROM THE LEAVES OF THE POISON IVY PLANT.

I began to experiment with homeopathic remedies for the illnesses of my two small children. The success rate was very high. Instead of wondering how it worked, I devoted myself to making it work even more successfully. When the treatments failed I went more deeply into the method of finding, for each case, the remedy that corresponded exactly to the illness.

I became fascinated by the magic of homeopathy and went on to take professional training and set up my own practice.

When the extreme pain of a physical injury fades from your body after taking the remedy *arnica*, when you see your child's high temperature fall after taking

ABOVE THE ARNICA PLANT IS USED TO MAKE A FIRST AID REMEDY THAT IS COMMONLY USED FOR BRUISING AND SHOCK. IT COMES IN TABLET AND CREAM FORM.

belladonna you start to make your beliefs fit this new reality.

People are rarely converted to homeopathy by an encounter with the theory. I certainly wasn't. But when it provides the solution in a time of dire need, or when it repeatedly does what it is not supposed to be able to do, then converts are made.

Even though science has not yet found an explanation, homeopathy still succeeds in treating all kinds of medical problems. But how does it work? Scientists may be near to finding the answer. The history of science is a history of expanding horizons; a continuous evolution of human understanding. At any point in time, it represents the limits of our vision rather than all there is to see. Larry Dossey, MD, writes:

'We continue to base our notions of health and illness, birth and death on visions of the world that have been transcended in our own time – the very physics that we look to has been modified in this century in all its major facets. Thus we find ourselves with models in medicine that are characterized not by accuracy, as we wished, but by obsolescence.'

The science that we are used to, the science that cannot explain homeopathy satisfactorily, is no longer the whole story. Our scientific understanding of the world is changing and the new theories are compatible with homeopathy. In the light of new scientific discoveries, the very dilute highly energized doses used in homeopathy are starting to make sense. In chaos and complexity theory very small changes in one part of a system can result in enormous changes elsewhere. This is what happens when a homeopathic remedy is taken.

These scientific revolutions are turning our understanding of the universe upside down. At the edges of our perceivable reality, that is at sub-microscopic levels and at astronomical levels, reality becomes unreliable and the rules start to change. It is because homeopathic medicines are taken to one of these edges, the subatomic level, and brought back again, that they are so revolutionary.

If a system of medicine were to be created in accordance with the principles of new physics, the result would be the reinvention of homeopathy. Chapter 3 will go a little further into the extraordinary support that is emerging for homeopathy from this physics. That 'plausible mode of action' may not be far away.

This book is intended as a practical guide to the use of homeopathic remedies in the home for the treatment of common minor ailments and injuries. Serious illness and injuries should always be referred to a qualified homeopath or medical practitioner as appropriate.

UNDERSTANDING HOMEOPATHY

CHAPTER ONE

Homeopathy is a natural system of treating all kinds of diseases. It is a subtle yet powerful system that works with the energies of life and produces genuine long-term cures in many complaints. It is based on holistic principles. This means that the medicine treats the whole person, not just one part or one disease.

THE FOUR BASIC PRINCIPLES

There are four principles on which homeopathy is based. The first two principles are shared with other holistic health treatments:

1   The treatment stimulates the body's *natural healing power*. (In homeopathy, this is called the *vital energy*.)
2   The treatment is *individually chosen* for each person.

The other two principles are unique to homeopathy:

3   The medicine is *similar* to the disease.
4   The doses used are minute and *potentized* (*see* p.16).

We will now look closely at these principles.

THE LAW OF SIMILARITY

The most important principle of homeopathy is the law of similarity. The word 'homeopathy' comes from two Greek words meaning 'similar suffering'. The law of similarity states: 'Whatever a medicine can cause in large doses in a healthy person, it can also cure in small doses in a sick person.' Or, put very simply, 'like cures like'.

For example, arsenic causes diarrhoea and great weakness, accompanied by restlessness and anxiety. Yet homeopathic doses of arsenic have cured many people of this same condition, whether the condition has been caused by food poisoning, colitis or cholera.

So the first step in developing a homeopathic remedy is to find out what it can cause. A homeopathic medicine is taken by healthy human volunteers in very small repeated doses to discover the set of symptoms it creates. (The medicines are never tested on animals.) These tests are called *provings*. They are double blind, which means that neither the supervisor nor the volunteers know what the substance is, nor which volunteers are getting placebos. As soon as changes in the provers' state of health begin, they stop taking the medicine before any permanent changes are produced. This ensures that the tests are safe. Each person's results are recorded and these records are then used to make up the *materia medica*, a description of what that medicine can cause. This is also called the remedy picture of that medicine.

To find the correct homeopathic remedy all the symptoms experienced by the sick person are recorded and compared with the remedy pictures until a similar one is found. When this remedy is taken in a potentized dose it stimulates the body to heal itself.

THE BODY'S NATURAL HEALING POWER

Homeopathic medicine does not treat the illness directly, but enables the human body to do the necessary healing for itself. The focus is on the patient rather than the disease. Because the remedy is similar to the disorder, it can stimulate the body to respond to the disease and cure it. Understanding this is crucial to the understanding of

AN EXAMPLE OF 'LIKE CURES LIKE'

CASE STUDY

A patient came to see me for homeopathic treatment because of panic attacks in the night that prevent him sleeping. He wakes suddenly at 1am, and is so restless he cannot stay in bed. He paces frantically around the house, and has such violent palpitations that he thinks he is about to die. He is anxious, restless, cold and trembling until 3 or 4am. Sometimes he can get to sleep better if he goes to a different bed. All these problems have been worse since the threat of redundancy, which has led to great anxiety about his financial affairs.

Here are some extracts from the proving of arsenic, *arsenicum album*, recorded by Dr Samuel Hahnemann, the founder of homeopathy, in his book *Materia Medica Pura*, published in 1830.

About 1am excessive anxiety. He can find rest in no place, continually changes his position in bed, will get out of one bed and into another, and lie now here, now there. He is cold, shivers and weeps, and thinks in his despair that nothing can help him, and he must die. Violent palpitation in the night. Rambling at night.

The remarkable similarity between the panic attacks of the patient and the experiences of the provers of *arsenicum album* mean that *arsenicum* is the remedy in this case.

13

RIGHT *ARSENICUM ALBUM*;
THE SYMPTOM PICTURE
IS CHARACTERIZED BY
RESTLESSNESS AND ANXIETY.

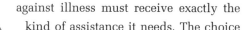

LEFT HOMEOPATHIC REMEDIES STIMULATE THE BODY'S NATURAL HEALING FORCE.

homeopathy as a whole. If you get a throat infection, your body has allowed the bacteria to multiply in your throat. The homeopathic remedy will stimulate your immune system to prevent this occurring, and so deal with the infection. Living organisms have the natural power to maintain health built into them. Every moment of our lives, our bodies are keeping us free of disease by constantly adjusting and balancing all the activities of the body. We adapt successfully to environmental changes and psychological stresses and defend ourselves against bacteria and viruses. We become ill only if our health maintenance system breaks down. Then we become susceptible to disease, and in order to be healthy again our defences need to be strengthened.

INDIVIDUAL TREATMENT

By treating the whole body, and its defences, homeopathy cures the illness. The medicine assists the forces fighting the illness, so it has to be compatible with those forces. Each person's struggle against illness must receive exactly the kind of assistance it needs. The choice

LEFT THE HOMEOPATH CAREFULLY FINDS OUT ABOUT THE WHOLE PERSON BY TAKING DETAILED CASE NOTES.

14

of medicine depends on the nature of the body's defences rather than the disease that is attacking it.

The way the body's defences are working is shown in the symptoms it produces in response to the disease. Two people with the same disease may not fight it in the same way and may therefore need different homeopathic treatment.

How does the homeopath tell which medicine each person's vital energy needs? By studying that person and their individual symptoms in detail. This is another central feature of homeopathy – the medicine is individually chosen for each patient. The choice of remedy will depend not only on the physical symptoms the person has, but also on his or her state of mind.

CASE STUDIES: INDIVIDUALIZED TREATMENT

Two children were brought to see me with ear infections.

In the first case the pain had begun at 3pm the previous day. The patient's right ear was hot and red, and she had a high fever.

In the second patient the ear had a discharge with an unpleasant odour, and the child could not stand any coldness or the slightest touch in the region of her ear. The child was hypersensitive and irritable.

These two children had the same medical condition, but they were reacting to it in different ways. The remedy indicated by the first set of symptoms was *belladonna*, and by the second, *hepar sulph.*

RIGHT IN HOMEOPATHY, PATIENTS WITH THE SAME PHYSICAL SYMPTOMS MAY RECEIVE DIFFERENT TREATMENTS.

15

POTENTIZATION

Nearly all homeopathic medicines are made from naturally occurring substances, mainly herbs and minerals. The medicines are diluted in a special way, stage by stage until they contain extremely small quantities of the original ingredient (*see* pp.34–37). At the same time they are shaken, or 'succussed', in a strictly controlled sequence. This process is called *potentization*. Paradoxically, the most dilute medicines have the most powerful healing effect.

THE HISTORY OF HOMEOPATHY

Although there are traces of homeopathic ideas right through medical history, homeopathy was only established as a medical system at the end of the 18th century by a German medical doctor called Samuel Hahnemann. Hahnemann had become thoroughly disenchanted with the medical treatments then available and began to conduct his own research. His first momentous discovery involved testing Peruvian bark (*cinchona officalis*), the source of quinine, which is used to treat malaria. Hahnemann discovered that when he took the bark, he got malaria symptoms. This was the first formal demonstration of the law of similarity.

After that discovery Hahnemann spent many years experimenting on himself and his students. They took repeated doses of many medicines and recorded their effects very accurately. They continued this proving of remedies over many years and built up a record of the symptoms produced by these medicines that, because of the law of similarity, they could also cure.

Whether by accident or inspiration, Hahnemann then made his second great discovery – potentization (*see* pp.34–37). He now had a method of making a medicine dilute enough to be safe, yet at the same time powerful enough to be effective.

By the early years of the 19th century the homeopathic method was established. Many of the treatments used at that time were rather barbaric and people welcomed the gentle way of homeopathy. Its use spread rapidly across Europe and to the United States. Treatments were extremely successful, and the system was adopted by Queen Victoria. Ever since then the British Royal Family has used and supported homeopathy.

One of homeopathy's most publicized successes of the 19th century was in the cholera epidemics of the 1850s. In the homeopathic hospital in London 16.4 per cent of cholera patients died; elsewhere it was 51.8 per cent.

However, the rise of homeopathy did not continue. Homeopathy went into a decline at the turn of the century as our present medical system grew stronger. Now, by contrast, homeopathy's fortunes are rising again as the limitations of conventional medicine become apparent. The demand for homeopathy is increasing dramatically and European manufacturers of homeopathic medicines regard Britain as a potential new market. Homeopathy is much more widely used in Europe. In France it is practised by 11,000 doctors and used by one third of the population.

17

YOUR VISIT TO A HOMEOPATH

When you visit a homeopath, the first part of the consultation will be similar to a visit to your doctor. You will describe your symptoms to the homeopath. However, the homeopath will also ask for apparently minor details of each symptom – such as the time of day when it is at its

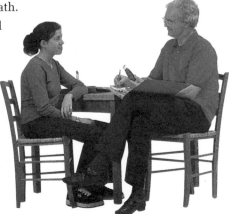

RIGHT A CONSULTATION WITH A HOMEOPATH INVOLVES ANSWERING MANY QUESTIONS. THIS IS TO BUILD UP A COMPLETE PATIENT PICTURE.

worst. Later there will be questions about you rather than your illness. For example, 'What are your favourite foods?' or 'do you have any phobias?' The homeopath is building up a complete picture of you as well as your illness. With this information and knowledge of the homeopathic remedies, the homeopath can categorize you as a certain homeopathic type, which is the particular homeopathic remedy that will restore your health (*see* Chapter 10, pp.106–113). You may be, for example, a *nux vomica* or a *pulsatilla*.

You will be given one medicine that will work on the whole of you – one medicine to stimulate healing even if you have several different complaints. The medicine is usually given in the form of small, white, almost tasteless tablets. You will also be given instructions on how to avoid anything that antidotes homeopathy (see pp.47–48).

You should then start to get better, though you may possibly feel slightly worse at the beginning of the treatment. (In emergencies the homeopathic remedy will work very quickly and without an 'aggravation'.) The remedy initiates a natural healing process so, in long-term complaints, the improvement is often gradual. On the other hand it is not confined only to the main illness. You should feel better in yourself, be able to cope with stress better, and your health generally should benefit.

Initial consultations usually last from 1–2 hours and cost from £30–50 in Britain. Further consultations cost less and are shorter and are rarely more frequent than once a month.

SOME COMMON MISCONCEPTIONS

Homeopathy relies on the placebo effect: It is sometimes suggested that homeopathic doses are so small that they cannot possibly work and that any benefits must be due to the placebo effect, or the healing effect of the long consultations. However, the effects of homeopathy cannot be explained away so easily as the remedies work on animals, babies and patients who are unconscious. In these latter cases the patient is not even aware of receiving any medicine so the placebo effect can be discounted. Also, there may well be no consultation at all, so that explanation collapses as well.

Homeopathy is a form of vaccination: The similarity between homeopathy and immunization is superficial. They both administer a substance similar to the disease and their effectiveness is based on arousing a reaction to that substance. Beyond that they are completely different. Immunizations mobilize the healing forces of the body only against one specific disease. Treatment with a homeopathic remedy raises the level of resistance to disease generally. The same immunization is given to everyone. In homeopathy, the treatment is individually chosen.

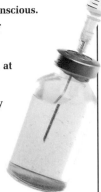

ABOVE VACCINATIONS DO NOT WORK IN THE SAME WAY AS HOMEOPATHY.

19

Homeopathy is unscientific: To explain how homeopathy is scientific, it is helpful to distinguish between a scientific method and a scientific explanation. Homeopathy is scientific in its method. The way of working out which remedy to give is systematic and consistent. The principles are clearly stated. The results can be assessed as in any scientific investigation.

To be scientific, the question of an explanation for these experimental results must be kept separate. Unbiased observation comes first. Only when we have the facts are we in a position to start explaining them properly. More experiments may then be needed. The controversial thing about homeopathy is that the scientific explanation is incomplete. But the experimental results are still valid and await a full explanation. The mechanics of the bumble bee's flight also await an explanation, but its journeys from flower to flower continue.

PROFESSIONAL HOMEOPATHS
AND HOMEOPATHIC DOCTORS

Once you have made the decision to have homeopathic treatment the next step is to find a properly trained homeopath. Although regulations in the British National Health Service have changed, most homeopathic treatment is still self-financed.

In Britain, homeopathy is practised by some conventional medical doctors and by professional homeopaths. Professional homeopaths are regulated by the Society of Homeopaths. They usually work in natural health clinics or their own consulting rooms, and sometimes in GP's surgeries.

The Society of Homeopaths publishes the Register of Homeopaths, which lists registered homeopaths in Britain. It also provides leaflets on homeopathy and other information. The Society is active in Britain and the rest of Europe in negotiating the future of professional homeopathy.

Generally speaking, professional homeopaths have more training in homeopathy and doctors have more training in medical science. Professional homeopaths tend to have longer consultations, although there are exceptions to this rule.

Doctors practising homeopathy are members of the Faculty of Homeopathy. The British Homeopathic Association provides information on homeopathy and lists of members of the Faculty.

Professional homeopaths and doctors are communicating more with each other, but there is still caution and mistrust on both sides.

Meanwhile, many people choose to have homeopathic treatment without their doctor knowing.

Taking Homeopathic Remedies with Orthodox Medicines

The question is often asked 'Do I have to stop taking my ordinary medicine when I start homeopathy?' Usually the answer is 'No'. Both the medicines will work normally, unaffected by each other. The main exceptions are antibiotics and oral steroids; these usually stop homeopathic remedies from working.

Once the homeopathy is working then most orthodox medicines can be stopped. This should usually be done gradually so the body has time to adjust. With some medicines the dose must be reduced very gradually. In some cases it is not safe to reduce the orthodox medication at all or only under medical supervision. For example, some treatments for high blood pressure and heart conditions. Considerations such as these sometimes, but very rarely, make homeopathic treatment impossible. Each case must be assessed on its own merit. If there is any doubt consult your doctor and homeopath.

21

What Homeopathy Can Do for You

Homeopathy is a safe natural system of medicine that does not have side-effects, although symptoms can sometimes get worse for a short time before they get better. The remedies are inexpensive, non-toxic and have a pleasant taste.

It is suitable for all age groups from newborn babies to the very old. It is excellent in pregnancy and childbirth.

RIGHT HOMEOPATHY HAS NO SIDE-EFFECTS AND MAY SAFELY BE USED BY PREGNANT WOMEN AND OTHER VULNERABLE GROUPS, SUCH AS CHILDREN.

Homeopathic treatment can be beneficial for the whole range of human diseases.

1   Infectious diseases from colds, sore throats and scabies to measles and pneumonia.

2   Diseases of all the major systems of the human body:

Heart and circulatory system, from high blood pressure and heart conditions to varicose veins;

Respiratory system, including croup and asthma;

Digestive system, from mouth ulcers to colitis;

Urinary and reproductive systems of both men and women, for example cystitis and kidney infections; and in women endometriosis and other gynaecological conditions, and in men enlarged prostate and impotence;

*Hormonal and nervous system*s, including meningitis, multiple sclerosis, thyroid disorders and all kinds of period problems;

Skin, for example eczema, psoriasis, acne, warts and verrucas;

Musculoskeletal system – the effectiveness of homeopathy in back problems is not often appreciated; it helps the body to adjust and align itself; apart from that it is very effective in sports injuries and all rheumatic and arthritic problems.

3 Being holistic, homeopathy also treats the mind and the emotions:

22

Mental problems – these may be minor, such as poor concentration in students or failing memory, or conditions arising from serious pathology such as Alzheimer's disease;

Emotional problems – all kinds of emotional problems respond very well to homeopathy – insomnia, anxiety, panic attacks, phobias, obsessions, manic-depression, violent and aggressive behaviour. Currently many parents are seeking homeopathic treatment for hyperactivity in children.

4   Homeopathy is a godsend in psychosomatic disorders, or for cases where it is not known whether there is a physical basis for the symptoms. This is because the remedy enables the vital energy of the patient to do whatever is necessary for healing, whether a mental or a physical change is needed.

5   One of the main benefits of homeopathy has not been mentioned. This is simply feeling better. Feeling better in yourself is often the first sign of a remedy working. An all-round improvement generally follows.

23

Homeopathy can also be used for first aid and for minor illnesses in the home. Equipped with a first aid kit of basic remedies and an introductory book such as this, you can learn how to treat yourself, your family and friends.

Homeopathy offers a safe natural way of treating most health problems. If you are looking for an alternative to the treatments you are familiar with, homeopathy is well worth investigation.

Many people come to homeopathy as a last resort, when they have not been able to find help elsewhere. Others first start using homeopathy as a preventative, before any serious illness develops. Often they have made an informed decision to follow natural methods as their first choice. They will use antibiotics or other orthodox treatments if their preferred choices fail. For them, orthodox treatments are the last resort. For some of us, this change in priorities comes when we become parents and want to give our children only natural medicines.

HEALTH AND DISEASE

CHAPTER TWO

Why is it that one person who has been exposed to the flu virus will go down with it when another will not? Why do some people develop meningitis when we all have the meningococcal bacteria present in our throats? Why does it prove fatal for one person whilst another receiving the same treatment recovers completely? The answer is that the severity of an infection depends not only on the virulence of the bacteria or virus but also on the ability of the immune system to combat the infection.

PREDISPOSITION TO DISEASE

Homeopaths call a flaw in the defence mechanism, or a constitutional weakness, a predisposition to disease. It is a tendency to, or an openness to, a certain kind of illness.

Predispositions are built into our constitutions by our inheritance and are influenced by environmental factors during our lives. Susceptibility to disease is a question of both nature and nurture. Predispositions can be triggered into actual illness by allergens, infection, stress, emotional and physical trauma, by bad diet and lifestyle, by aging and the developmental stages of life such as teething, puberty and menopause, and by many other factors.

CASE STUDY: PREDISPOSITION TO DISEASE

A two-year-old girl became emotionally insecure and very clingy after her mother was away from home for a week. She then caught chicken pox. After this she developed eczema.

This shows how the predisposition to eczema was activated by external influences. The separation and the chicken pox triggered changes in her level of health. After taking *pulsatilla*, her constitutional remedy, she soon became herself again and her eczema disappeared.

VITAL ENERGY

During the course of every seven year period, our entire physical body is replaced. After this time not a single molecule of the previous body remains. This includes the DNA molecules. Yet no one would deny that we are the same human being. Clearly the continuity does not come from the physical substance. The continuity is provided by an organizing principle, a formative energy that controls and maintains the human body. This formative energy is at work every moment energizing the processes of life – for example, it guides the transformation of our food into our bodily structure. Besides the daily miracle of turning our breakfast into bone tissue, this blueprint of human individuality keeps all the systems of the human body working in harmony together. The maintenance of this human form and the maintenance of health are one and the same process. Illness occurs if this process breaks down. Disease starts as a disorder of life energy, not of physical substance. A person is a unified whole with inbuilt healing capabilities – these simply need activating. The role of vital energy is crucial.

This vital energy, which is a central principle of homeopathy, has many names. Hippocrates called it 'the healing force of nature',

25

alchemists called it 'vital fluid'. In acupuncture it is *chi*, in yoga, *prana*. Like magnetism and electricity and all forms of energy, it cannot be seen but is clearly detectable by its effects. Well-known homeopath George Vithoulas writes:

> 'What occurs at the moment of death? The organism is structurally intact, cells are busily functioning, chemical reactions are still proceeding, yet a sudden change occurs and the body begins to decompose! Reflection upon this thought makes the concept of vital forces not only understandable, but appealing.'

The life force that departs at death is the difference between living tissue and dead tissue. It inhabits and animates our living bodies, protecting living tissue from disintegration and decay. To illustrate this, consider just one of the millions of self-regulating and self-healing activities that our bodies perform. If an infection develops in a wound then the immune system springs into action. Inflammation brings white blood cells to the wound to eliminate the invaders. These cells are transported from the bone marrow via the circulatory system. The 'intelligence system' of the body may cause the hypothalamus to adjust its thermostat to produce a high temperature. This accelerates body activity generally and increases antibody production. One simple self-regulating activity can involve many body systems. Our self-healing systems are part of our anatomy and physiology. The normal processes of life and the maintenance of health are totally integrated.

Vital energy invisibly permeates our physical bodies, working without our conscious involvement. It is creative, formative and intelligent. Homeopaths believe that it is responsible for the state of our health. In health this vibrant energy is strong and harmonious. When this energy is weak or out of balance, we become ill. In other words, if our health breaks down it is because our vital energy has failed, allowing disorder to creep in where the harmonious forces of life are not in control. Strong vital energy enables us and our bodies to bounce back to health when we come up against things that can trigger disease. The 'inflatable castles' that our children enjoy always have leaks, but as long as the motor is powerful, the castle will retain its bounce. Good vital energy is like that motor – it compensates for the inevitable daily demands on our bodies and minds and gives us some bounce to spare. Without this vitality disease can move into the vacuum and take over. Our vital energy needs to be enhanced, unblocked, strengthened, harmonized, or one could almost say, re-educated or reprogrammed.

THE HOLISTIC VIEW OF HEALTH

Body and mind are a continuum – they cannot be separated and they influence each other. The sight of a lion produces adrenalin, the thought of a good meal produces digestive enzymes. Consciousness and substance are indivisibly linked in a living human organism. The psychologist C G Jung describes how the lower regions of the mind blend into the physical body:

'The deep "layers" of the psyche lose their individual uniqueness as they retreat further and further into darkness. "Lower down", that is to say as they approach the autonomous functional systems, they... are... extinguished in the body's materiality, i.e. in chemical substance.'

We must regard a human being as a unified mind-body system. The health of the mind or the body is dependent on the health of the whole person. A sickness in one part of the human being is a sickness of the whole.

This is the philosophy of holism applied to health and disease – the whole is greater than the sum of the parts. The essence of a human being cannot be found in any one part, not in body, mind, cell

27

SCIENTIFIC CONFIRMATION OF VITAL ENERGY

• Kirlian Photography. This special photographic technique shows how all objects, living or non-living, are surrounded by energy fields. Bright patterns are seen around a healthy person. When the person is ill, the patterns seen in Kirlian photographs become weaker and more chaotic.

• Relativity. The most famous equation in science is Einstein's $E=mc^2$. This small but highly important equation states that energy and matter can be interchangeable. So the physical matter of our bodies is not the fixed foundation of our existence; we must concede a role to energy in our understanding of substance and therefore of disease.

• New Physics. Physicists now take this further. In order to explain the subatomic world they have been forced to conclude that another unknown level of reality exists. The subatomic particles of physical matter are constantly appearing out of, and disappearing back into, this other level of existence. The old theories of solid substance have dematerialized between our fingers. All things, including human beings, are the unfolded parts of a quantum sea of potential existence. Therefore, our physical bodies depend for their existence upon an invisible backcloth of potentiality. There is a similar relationship between health and vital energy. Vital energy is the invisible backcloth that determines our health.

• The Memory Of Water. Research by the famous French immunologist Jacques Benveniste (published in the scientific journal *Nature*) has shown that homeopathic remedies leave an energy pattern in the water used to dilute them. In effect, water has a memory. Another intriguing example of this is found in snowflakes. All snowflakes have their own unique crystal structure, despite their astronomical numbers. Yet, melted snowflakes that have been frozen again resume the same original crystal shape.

or gene, nor indeed in all the parts together. It is something more than all the constituent parts. Plato, the Ancient Greek philosopher, said:

'The cure of the part should not be attempted without treatment of the whole. No attempt should be made to cure the body without the soul, and if the head and body are to be healthy you must begin by curing the mind.'

SELF-HEALING SYSTEMS

Our integral self-healing systems provide adjustments and responses to constant changes in our environments and our lives. The responses are unified through many systems and levels of organization. Homeopathy is one way of strengthening your system and helping to achieve a natural balance, both emotionally and physically. Emotional stress directly affects the physical body. The reverse also holds – our psychological state is affected by our bodies. The whole system becomes stronger when homeopathic treatment works.

We can also help our vital energy to keep us healthy by finding the problems in our lives that are draining it – conflicts in relationships, frustrations at work, negative emotions, damaging patterns of behaviour. All these can consume our precious vitality so that there is less available to maintain good health. Then our predispositions are uncovered and illness develops. By giving positive attention to all aspects of our lives and finding ways of working through the problems, we put less strain on ourselves.

If you are at ease with yourself this will help to keep your body free of 'dis-ease'. 'Dis-ease' is being out of balance in mind and body – the harmony of the whole organism is disturbed.

Whatever constitution you have, weak or strong, you can make the best of your endowment by healthy living. This means eating fresh natural foods and not burdening your body too much with tobacco and alcohol, or any other unhealthy props. When we understand ourselves in the way described here then we will prefer treatments that respect our bodies as self-healing systems. We are intricate and beautiful beings; medicines can work with the natural forces that maintain our health. Medicines should also respect our individual patterns of illness. They should go to the core of the problem, which is the core of ourselves. The whole, which is something more than all the parts, must be healed. Homeopathy is one of the medical systems that can give these benefits.

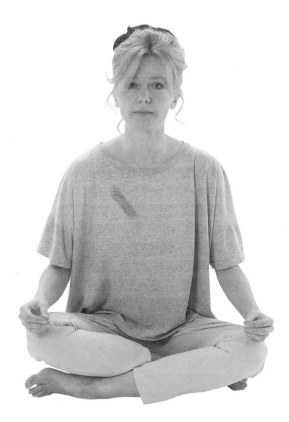

ABOVE WE MUST TREAT OUR BODIES WITH RESPECT IF WE WISH TO STAY HEALTHY IN BOTH BODY AND MIND.

HOW HOMEOPATHY WORKS

CHAPTER THREE

Homeopathy works because its two main pillars, *the law of similarity* and *potentization*, complement each other. Together they make up the homeopathic system – a system of medicine that can make a tremendous contribution to health care. However, before this can happen patients and medical practitioners need a better understanding of how homeopathy works. This chapter starts with a look at how orthodox medicines work and this, in turn, highlights the different approach taken in homeopathic medicine.

THE ALLOPATHIC VERSUS THE HOMEOPATHIC APPROACH

Allopathic treatment involves inducing an opposite effect to that produced by the disease. For example, when we take an anti-inflammatory drug for an arthritic hip its effect is to alter the biochemistry of the body. The presence

LEFT ORTHODOX DRUGS WORK ON THE DISEASE ITSELF BUT DO LITTLE TO PREVENT THE DISEASE OCCURRING IN THE FIRST PLACE.

of the drug neutralizes the inflammation, and the hip will therefore feel better. When we take a sleeping tablet, we are swallowing chemicals that induce sleep. The active ingredient enters our internal chemical laboratory and, until it is dispersed, corrects the imbalance that is causing insomnia.

In both these examples the medication can be repeated as necessary to maintain the right biochemical levels.

Homeopaths, by contrast, would ask why is there this inflammation of the hip in the first place? It is not only unnecessary – because there is no injury to repair or foreign body to expel – it is positively harmful. The body is making a mistake – it is malfunctioning.

ABOVE HOMEOPATHY TREATS THE BODY AS AN INTELLIGENT SELF-REGULATING SYSTEM THAT HEALS ITSELF IF GIVEN THE RIGHT IMPETUS.

The cause of the disease is not in the hip, nor even in the inflammatory process, which is an essential part of the defence mechanism. The cause is in the self-regulating system that initiates the misplaced inflammation. In the case of insomnia, the problem is caused by the patient's metabolism having become stuck in the waking mode.

In the allopathic medical treatment described above, the problem is relieved temporarily by each dose of medication. However, the body is still trying to produce the inflammation. Homeopathic treatment works to assist the body's own self-regulatory system. Instead of targeting the end product of the malfunction, i.e. the inflammation, it works to correct the process at its source so that the body no longer produces the inflammation.

Homeopathic medicine acts on the self-regulating system of the body rather than directly on the physical level. It reprogrammes this system to bring it back to a normal healthy pattern. In effect, it would point out to the body its mistake. It treats the body as an intelligent self-governing organization.

Homeopaths suggest that this vital regulatory system can work properly if given the right stimulus. This right stimulus is a mimic of the disease that then produces a healing response from the vital energy. We tend to underestimate the wisdom of the body. Most illnesses are healed without any medicine at all. When they are not, the vital energy only needs the right encouragement. Homeopathic remedies work with the natural efforts of the body, guiding them in the right direction.

This is why the medicine given in homeopathic treatment is similar to the disease. The homeopathic remedy acts as a version of the disorder that the human organism responds to. The response will be the reorganization that is needed to re-establish health. The organism's innate healing intelligence will do whatever is necessary.

The law of similarity works by drawing a response from the body's own healing abilities. The homeopathic remedy produces a reaction from the creative life energy hidden within each of us.

For example, you have a cup of coffee when you need to be alert and motivated, quick-thinking and resourceful. A material dose of *coffea tosta*, an infusion of ground roast coffee beans, can produce that state for you.

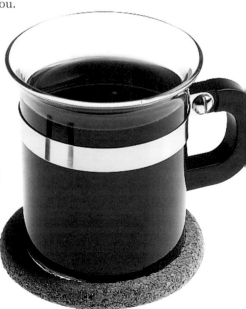

But what should you do if you are in that state and do not want to be? Perhaps you have been to a very intense meeting or a very exciting party one evening and afterwards cannot get to sleep.

In these circumstances a homeopathic dose of *coffea tosta* will neutralize this state and bring peace and rest.

RIGHT CAFFEINE STIMULATES THE BODY AND MIND. BY CONTRAST, *COFFEA*, THE REMEDY MADE FROM COFFEE BEANS, QUIETENS AN OVEREXCITED STATE.

33

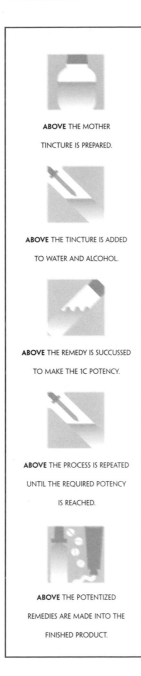

ABOVE THE MOTHER
TINCTURE IS PREPARED.

ABOVE THE TINCTURE IS ADDED
TO WATER AND ALCOHOL.

ABOVE THE REMEDY IS SUCCUSSED
TO MAKE THE 1C POTENCY.

ABOVE THE PROCESS IS REPEATED
UNTIL THE REQUIRED POTENCY
IS REACHED.

ABOVE THE POTENTIZED
REMEDIES ARE MADE INTO THE
FINISHED PRODUCT.

POTENTIZATION

Potentizing a medicine is not only a method of diluting it to reduce side-effects. It achieves much more than this – it gives it special properties. The therapeutic effect is increased while the toxic effect is reduced. Paradoxically, the process also increases the strength of the medicine for a person who needs it. For the person whose health problems correspond to that medicine, one dose will have a powerful beneficial effect. For others for whom it is not the right remedy, many doses will do nothing. For example, the remedy *phosphorus* cured one patient of nosebleeds. A relative who suffered from the same problem treated himself for several weeks with a whole bottle of *phosphorus* tablets. This had no effect on him at all – it is the quality of similarity that triggers the therapeutic effect, not the quantity of doses.

As the remedies are repeatedly diluted, they are also succussed, that is, they are shaken in a predetermined way a set number of times. On the most commonly used scale of potencies, the medicine is diluted one part in 100 parts of a water/alcohol mixture, and then shaken 50 times. This process of dilution by 100 is repeated five times more to produce the sixth potency on the centesimal scale (measured in units of dilution by 100).

This potency is referred to as 6c. The potency of the remedy increases with dilution, and 6c is a low potency. Repetition of the dilution 30 times yields the 30th potency, which is still quite low. The 200th, 1,000th and 10,000th potencies are high potencies.

PREPARATION OF A HOMEOPATHIC REMEDY: *SILICA*

I have chosen *silica* as an example because it shows how an insoluble substance can be turned into a homeopathic remedy. The starting point is flint, one of the many natural forms of silicon dioxide. The flint is first ground into a powder. This is then ground in a mortar and pestle with lactose for three hours. After that it can be potentized in the same way as a soluble substance. One part of this preparation is mixed with 99 parts of alcohol and succussed. Each repetition of this process raises the potency one step higher.

RIGHT A PESTLE AND MORTAR ARE USED TO GRIND UP THE RAW MATERIALS USED IN THE PREPARATION OF HOMEOPATHIC MEDICINES.

This apparently straightforward method takes us through the physical structure of the substance into its underlying energy field. We know beyond doubt from modern physics that the particles that make up physical matter are concentrations of energy that appear and disappear – the particles appear briefly out of a sea of quantum energy and soon disappear back into it. Matter is merely the visible part of an energy field. This is not overenthusiastic wishful thinking but demonstrable fact. Given the right conditions, science has shown that matter and energy are interchangeable. Potentization is a method of making the energy that is hidden in matter available.

For example, the *silica* sample in the box above could provide enough high potency tablets to treat thousands of people. In some rare cases, remedies have been made by taking the life of an animal. However, one life is enough simply because the remedies are so dilute. For example the remedy *tarentula* was made from a spider killed 100 years ago. Even now all preparations of this remedy originate from that one spider.

THE EFFECTIVENESS OF VERY HIGH DILUTIONS

• In biology, the Arndt-Schultz law states that very strong stimuli are harmful to living organisms whereas very small ones are beneficial. Small stimuli activate our responses.

• There are many instances of animals being affected by extremely small concentrations of hormones, enzymes and other substances. For example, insects are attracted by pheromones from the opposite sex at huge distances. In the sea, sharks can detect extraordinarily small amounts of blood.

• Inside the human body concentrations of thyroid hormone of one part in 10,000 parts of blood lead to marked changes in metabolic processes.

• The human sense of smell can detect the substance mercaptan when there is only one part present in 500,000,000,000 parts of air. The Appendix (*see* p.115) gives a selection of all the laboratory tests that have been done on the effects of homeopathic potencies on enzymes, blood antibodies, plant growth rates, etc. The scientific evidence shows that the potencies have definite effects.

IN CONCLUSION

Chaos theory and other developments in scientific thinking have shown that we can revolutionize our understanding of how the universe works. Can we take this revolution far enough to make homeopathy scientifically acceptable?

Science is closer than we might think to providing an explanation for how homeopathy works. The parallels between long-established homeopathic principles and recent scientific discoveries are gratifying for homeopaths and open up exciting possibilities for further research.

There is a well-known example that illustrates chaos theory. The flap of a butterfly's wing in Australia can lead, via a long chain of increasing results, to a tornado in America. When a system is on the point of changing, it takes very little to push it over the brink. A tiny change can trigger a gigantic change in a charged system but the small push must be in the direction the system is trying to go. This is how a very small dose of a medicine similar to the disease can bring about healing.

Physicist David Bohm writes:

'Matter as we know it is a small "quantized" wave-like excitation on top of this background [of energy]. Further developments in physics may make it possible to probe the above mentioned background in a more direct way.'

Perhaps potentization is a method of probing that releases from matter its medical powers.

The most exciting thing about the many scientific revelations of recent years is the increased reverence for nature that scientists are developing. After four billion years of research and development, nature has produced solutions to countless problems whose existence has not even occurred to us. In this new atmosphere of wonderment, homeopathy becomes more credible. Our bodies have subtleties and complexities that we know nothing about. Many processes of life are beyond our understanding. Homeopathic medicines give us a means of healing that respects and enhances this creation that is beyond our understanding.

VISITING A
HOMEOPATH

CHAPTER FOUR

Consulting a homeopath may be a new experience for you and it helps to know what is involved before you start (*see* pp.17–18). The consultation with the homeopath will be spent compiling a full profile of you and your illness from a homeopathic perspective. In theory, this can be divided into three stages:

1   The first stage is when you describe your problems to the homeopath. The homeopath may well encourage you to say more. You should tell him or her anything that is troubling you – emotional difficulties or anything else that is not going well in your life – as well as physical complaints.

2   Then the homeopath will want more details of all your problems. You may be asked direct and specific questions at this stage. You may be asked how and when each problem started and developed, what triggers or influences each symptom, how each pain feels, and so on.

LEFT BY ANSWERING ANY QUESTIONS IN AS MUCH DETAIL AS POSSIBLE,
YOU WILL HELP YOUR HOMEOPATH TO BUILD UP A
COMPLETE PROFILE OF YOU.

3 The third stage is where the homeopath finds out more about you by asking the characteristic homeopathic questions. For example, what foods do you strongly like or dislike? How are you affected by the seasons and different weather conditions? How well do you sleep? What are you afraid of? When do you get nervous? What do you worry about? How sociable are you? What experiences have had a deep effect on you? The answers will give the homeopath an impression of your personality type and your outlook on life. However, don't stick strictly to the questions – use them as springboards to help you talk about yourself. Sometimes patients will tell homeopaths things they have never told anyone else. Be honest and open – this will help the homeopath find the right remedy for you.

You may start to think that the homeopath believes your illness to be psychosomatic. This is not so, but homeopaths have found that a person's state of mind is a trustworthy guide to finding the remedy that will heal both body and mind.

The homeopath will be scrutinizing you carefully, without being judgmental – the aim is to understand you as an individual. Information such as the diagnosis, test results, medical history, and the treatment you are already receiving is needed by the homeopath. However, this is not important in the choice of remedy, so it is not the main concern of the consultation. Homeopaths are like detectives tracking down clues; they do not want to miss one – that one clue could be the key to the whole case.

39

RIGHT THE BEHAVIOUR AND MOOD OF THE PATIENT WILL BE OBSERVED CLOSELY DURING THE CONSULTATION.

CHOOSING A HOMEOPATH

Choosing who to go to with your health problems should be a careful and informed decision.

When you look for a homeopath, bear the following considerations in mind:

• Qualifications. You may want to check the homeopath's qualifications by speaking to them personally, or by contacting the relevant professional body (*see*, p.20 and Useful Addresses, p.122).

• Reputation. Take into account reports you have heard in your area, bearing in mind that no homeopath is going to be able to cure every case.

• Professionalism. Your homeopath should have a professional way of working, including the following – a suitable place of work, an organized appointments system, reasonable accessibility for enquiries and emergencies, proper storage for remedies and patient case files, assurance of confidentiality and a commitment to the work of healing.

• Your homeopath should be someone you can get on with and in whom you have confidence. Do you want to see a man or a woman? Do you want to meet the homeopath briefly and find out if you feel comfortable with him or her before committing yourself? Do you want to check beforehand that your problems can be helped by homeopathy? You should be able to telephone and ask any questions you may have. Many homeopaths will offer a short introductory appointment either free of charge or for a small fee.

40

RIGHT EMPATHY BETWEEN PATIENT AND

HOMEOPATH IS VITAL.

It is not always easy for the patient to understand what the homeopath needs to know. Patients get concerned that they are giving their homeopath the wrong kind of information. Here are some guidelines to help you:

• Try to simply supply information. For instance, state the time of day when you feel a certain pain or state of mind, rather than explaining why you should experience it at that particular time. Noticing that eating cheese stops you sleeping is important, or saying that when you cannot sleep you start to fear that you have cancer is important. The homeopath does not interpret or explain such observations but just takes note of them.

• Tell the truth about yourself, including your difficult side, such as having a bad temper or being intolerant of certain things. The homeopath needs to know anything you are sensitive to. It may be helpful to mention the comments other people make about you.

Your deepest fears and secrets are very important in the choice of remedy. These things are not silly or shameful. The homeopath will have listened to such sensitive issues many times before, and mentioning them is important.

Some people enjoy unburdening themselves in this way. For others it may be an invasion of personal space or a difficult confession. Homeopaths acknowledge that some issues may be too painful to uncover and will respect your wishes.

Equally, do not feel put off if you have no deep inner struggles – there will still be other things to talk about.

THE ROLE OF THE HOMEOPATH

The homeopath's first role is 'active listening'. This involves helping the patient to give the information that is needed. Patients may at times need gentle encouragement to express themselves. The aim of the homeopath is to form a well-rounded 'portrait in words' of his or her patient.

41

During this process you may be able to sense the homeopath's mind working, absorbing the information you are giving and putting it into some kind of order. For the homeopath, each case is a jigsaw puzzle that can be assembled in many ways. He or she will try one way and get a picture that resembles, perhaps, the remedy *pulsatilla*. Putting the symptoms into a different pattern may produce a better likeness of the remedy *staphysagria*. Then a certain feature of the case may reveal a striking image of the remedy *cuprum*. Insight, knowledge of *materia medica* and homeopathic skills are working together here on the main challenge in homeopathy.

Each case is unique. The homeopath is reading the symptoms of the patient. Each symptom and characteristic of the person is a clue in this detective work.

When the homeopath has enough clues he or she can understand the pattern lying behind the physical and psychological state and categorize each person as one of a hundred or more homeopathic types. You may have to wait a few days before the homeopath has finished working out the remedy you need.

ASSESSING THE TREATMENT

After taking the medicine according to the instructions, several weeks will elapse before your next appointment. During that time you should continue to avoid anything that might antidote the treatment. If the treatment is going well you will start to understand the homeopathic healing process. If you have any questions telephone the homeopath.

The healing process has its own logic and sequence. The cure proceeds from within the body outwards and may take some time to reach the main problems. Very often patients will say 'I felt better in myself quite quickly. My main problem is not much better really, but I am coping with it and it is not affecting my life so much. It was worse for a couple of days at first.'

This is an excellent reaction to the treatment and must be allowed to unfold without interference. You can now feel confident that your illness is being cured at a deep level and you will soon experience a long period of much improved health.

At the second visit you should report all the changes you have noticed. Keeping notes can be helpful but once a week is enough to record the overall trends. You will be asked about all the problems you mentioned in the first consultation so that the process of cure can be mapped. Sometimes, gradual changes only become apparent at this stage and after the follow-up consultation you realize how much has changed. Patience is sometimes needed at this point. Some severe and long-standing conditions will get better very slowly and may have to get worse at first. Good homeopathic treatment can transform your health and your life but this may take some time. Patience will also be needed if the treatment is not working. The homeopath will then need to reconsider everything, and give you a new remedy.

43

The Consultation as a Learning Experience

Having homeopathic treatment can be a learning experience in several ways:
• You may learn something about yourself or acknowledge new facets of yourself as a result of the consultation or the changes you feel after the treatment.
• The in-depth interview and the stages of recovery are an education in the relationship of disease to human nature.
• Above all, if you are intending to study homeopathy, then experiencing it personally is an unrivalled foundation for your developing knowledge. However, students of homeopathy and homeopaths themselves can sometimes be the worst patients because they see themselves in terms of all the different remedies. This affects how they describe themselves in the consultation.

YOUR HOME REMEDY KIT

CHAPTER FIVE

Homeopathic remedies are becoming more easily available in health food stores and pharmacies. For a wider selection of remedies and potencies you can order from a specialist pharmacy (*see* Useful Addresses, p.122). Sets of remedies can be supplied in their own carrying cases. It is important to have a conventional first-aid kit and know conventional first-aid techniques, such as mouth-to-mouth resuscitation – this can be learned at a first-aid course. Keep a manual and bandages with your remedies and make sure you have a good family health handbook.

THE FIRST-AID KIT

The introduction to homeopathy for many people is *arnica*, which is often needed in accidents and injuries. Therefore, it makes sense to start with *arnica* and expand your kit as funds allow.

The following remedies will cover most injuries and accidents, including bites, stings and burns:

Arnica, bryonia, calendula, cantharis, hypericum, ledum, ruta and *rhus tox. Bellis perennis, symphytum, staphysagria* and *urtica* are needed less often but should be added if possible.

ABOVE SOME HOMEOPATHIC REMEDIES ARE AVAILABLE IN CREAM FORM FOR EXTERNAL USE. THESE MAY BE USED IN THE FIRST AID TREAMENT OF CUTS AND GRAZES.

Calendula or *hypericulum/calendula* cream for cuts and grazes and a cream for minor burns would also be useful. Rescue Remedy or Five Flower Remedy, which are combinations of flower remedies introduced by Dr Edward Bach, are helpful in any shock or stress.

THE BASIC HOME REMEDY KIT
The next step is to build up a kit of the remedies most often needed for common illnesses:

Aconite, apis mellifica, arsenicum album, belladonna, chamomilla, ferrum phosphorica, gelsemium, ignatia, lachesis, lycopodium, mercury, nux vomica, phosphorus, pulsatilla, rhus tox., silica, sulphur, staphysagria.

Other remedies are used less often and can be added individually as needed.

45

RIGHT KEEP YOUR REMEDIES AWAY FROM DIRECT LIGHT. STORE IN CLEARLY LABELLED BOTTLES AND ONLY OPEN THEM WHEN NECESSARY.

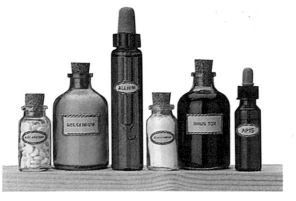

STORING THE MEDICINES

Properly stored homeopathic remedies will last indefinitely. Only open the bottle you need, and for the shortest possible time. Do not put tablets back into the bottles once they have been taken out. Store your remedies in a cool dark place away from computer and television screens and other electromagnetic fields.

How to Give
Homeopathic Medicines

Homeopathic tablets should never be touched, except by the patient just before they are taken. To take one, the patient should put it onto his or her clean hand or into something such as a clean dry spoon, or into the cap of the remedy bottle, and put it straight into the mouth. The tablets should not be swallowed but allowed to dissolve under the tongue. This may take a few seconds or half an hour depending on the density of the tablet.

The tablets are made of lactose – sugar of milk. However, anyone who is lactose intolerant of even small quantities can take the remedies in liquid form.

For babies, if you cannot get the remedy as a liquid or as small granules, then crush a tablet into a powder between two clean dry spoons. This way the baby will not be able to spit out the tablet or choke on it.

Giving remedies to animals sometimes requires ingenuity. Tablets crushed between two clean dry spoons into a powder can sometimes be put into the mouths of larger animals such as horses. For cats and dogs I usually dissolve several crushed tablets in a little milk or water. Otherwise follow the same procedures as for humans.

The time of day you take the tablet does not matter, but you must have nothing by mouth for half an hour before and after taking it – do

46

LEFT AVOID TOUCHING THE REMEDY. TIP THE TABLET INTO THE CONTAINER LID AND PUT STRAIGHT INTO THE MOUTH.

not drink, eat, smoke, clean your teeth and so on. After a strong curry or other food with a persistent taste you may have to wait even longer for the taste to disperse. However, this time limit can be reduced to a few minutes if it is not possible to wait longer, especially if only water is being taken.

ANTIDOTES TO HOMEOPATHIC TREATMENT

While taking homeopathic treatment you should avoid having anything that stops the treatment working. In the case of chronic illness this should be for as long as the benefit continues. Treatment for acute illness cannot be antidoted once the patient is better.

47

Some of the strongest antidotes are things containing camphor, eucalyptus and menthol. The damage is done by inhaling the vapour, so just smelling these things can antidote. Olbas oil, Vick, Carvol, Deep-Heat, and many other inhalants, muscle relaxants, lip salves and even mothballs must be strictly avoided. Recreational drugs also antidote homeopathy.

In addition, avoid drinking coffee. Even a few sips have been known to antidote on occasions. Weak instant de-caffeinated coffee and coffee cake or chocolates do not usually cause problems.

RIGHT AVOID SMELLING ANY SUBSTANCES THAT CONTAIN CAMPHOR, EUCALYPTUS OR MENTHOL. VAPOURS FROM THESE PRODUCTS MAY ANTIDOTE THE HOMEOPATHIC REMEDY.

Most conventional medicines can be taken alongside homeopathic treatment – there will be no interference in either direction. (There may, however, be some confusion afterwards about which treatment has worked.)

The exceptions to this are antibiotic tablets, steroid tablets, immunizations and anaesthetics of any kind, even local ones, and dental anaesthetics. If possible plan immunizations and dental work that requires an anaesthetic before, or at least two months after, homeopathic treatment for long-term problems. Once a patient has stopped taking antibiotic or steroid tablets, homeopathic treatment can begin within two days. Remember that steroids and some other medicines can be discontinued only with medical supervision.

Be wary of treating anyone who is having, or has recently had, homeopathic treatment for long-term health problems. Giving any homeopathic remedies at this stage could interfere with the treatment. Contact the homeopath concerned first.

Emotional shocks and traumas can also sometimes antidote homeopathic treatment.

You may think you have antidoted your remedy, but a few days later you start to get better again. In treating chronic complaints it is important to wait for two weeks before repeating the remedy, to see if it really has been antidoted.

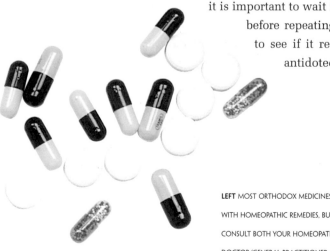

LEFT MOST ORTHODOX MEDICINES CAN BE TAKEN WITH HOMEOPATHIC REMEDIES, BUT IF IN DOUBT CONSULT BOTH YOUR HOMEOPATH AND DOCTOR/GENERAL PRACTITIONER.

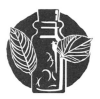

BEFORE YOU BEGIN

CHAPTER SIX

irst you need to know some definitions. An acute illness is a short-term illness such as a cold, flu, pneumonia etc. It is something you normally recover from after a few days (or a few weeks with some of the more severe ones). A chronic illness is one that tends to continue long-term and to get worse, such as eczema, irritable bowel syndrome and heart disease. *This book deals mainly with acute illnesses.*

THE STAGES OF
HOMEOPATHIC TREATMENT

There are five essential stages in all homeopathic treatment. The stages may seem rather obvious but remembering this sequence, especially during a health crisis, will help you to get the very best out of homeopathy.

1 *Decide whether it is appropriate for you to give homeopathic treatment.*

2 *Take the case.* This means recording all the information about the illness and the patient. This may range from one sentence such as 'I hit my finger with a

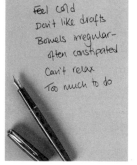

RIGHT RECORD PHYSICAL AND EMOTIONAL SYMPTOMS.

hammer and it's gone blue and it hurts' to several pages of notes. Only when this is complete should you go on to step three.

3   *Analyse the case.* To organize the case notes make a list of the symptoms. From this you will be able to work out the remedy.

4   *Give the remedy.* Decide which of the categories (from emergency to chronic) described on pp.51–53 and 108–109 fits your case. Each category has its own guidance on dosage etc.

5   *Assess the reaction.* Record the patient's reaction to the remedy and decide whether further treatment is needed. Keep all the records of each patient you treat as this may help with future treatment. (Sometimes subsequent illnesses will need the same homeopathic remedy.)

Conducting a homeopathic consultation and selecting the remedy required are skills that develop with experience. You will know a little already if you have been to a homeopath. If you also have the chance to observe a homeopath at work, do so. There is nothing better than live experience. You can then study the notes and work out possible remedies without actually giving them, and learn a lot that way. Also try to practise on your friends.

WHEN IS IT APPROPRIATE TO GIVE HOMEOPATHIC TREATMENT?

When you begin to use the remedies for yourself, family and friends, start with the conditions that are easiest to treat, such as minor injuries. As you gain knowledge and confidence go on to more difficult problems. It is not unusual to have a period of beginner's luck at first, and then become overenthusiastic, wanting to

LEFT NOSEBLEEDS AND OTHER SIMPLE MINOR COMPLAINTS CAN SAFELY BE TREATED BY THE INEXPERIENCED HOMEOPATHIC PRACTITIONER.

treat everyone and everything. Next comes a phase of disappointment when none of the remedies you give seem to work. This is an initiation into the enduring work of homeopathy and the dedication required to keep studying human nature and disease in the light of homeopathic knowledge. The next phase is one of maturity, where you are less eager to show everyone that homeopathy can save the world, but are getting a consistent level of success. By now you will also be aware that you cannot rush up to every accident you witness and administer *arnica*!

As a beginner in homeopathy the first question to ask yourself when someone needs help is 'Am I capable of taking this patient on?' If you read the three sections below and the fourth on pp. 108–109, you will be able to categorize your case and then follow the guidelines for that category.

In categories one and two contact the emergency services, doctor or homeopath first before thinking about homeopathic treatment. Trying homeopathic remedies while waiting for the doctor to arrive can do no harm. In category three there is less urgency and you can experiment more with homeopathy.

How to Use Homeopathic Remedies

1: EMERGENCY ACUTE ILLNESSES

The illness is life-threatening and help is needed urgently. Examples are some injuries, infections, asthma attacks and bleeding, etc.

Professional Help: Make sure the ambulance is on its way and you have given whatever practical assistance you can. You can then give homeopathic treatment yourself while you are waiting, if appropriate, or contact a homeopath.

Dose: One tablet of low potency every 10 seconds for three doses. One dose of one tablet of potency 30 or higher.

Assessment: These cases require fast action and the right remedy will act within seconds in the most urgent cases. If there is no effect go on to a different remedy.

Also, the effect of one tablet may soon be exhausted so frequent repetitions may be required. You may need to give one tablet of a low potency as often as every few seconds. Even potencies of 30 and over may need repetition every few minutes to maintain the effect.

2: SEVERE ACUTE ILLNESSES

Although not immediately life-threatening, the illness is still serious. Examples include some cases of pneumonia, infections, injuries.

Professional Help: The doctor should be called and also the homeopath, if appropriate. If homeopathy is used then it must be effective quickly. Otherwise antibiotics or other conventional treatment will be necessary.

Dose: One tablet of low potency every three minutes for three doses. One dose of potency 30 or higher.

Assessment: Wait for between 30 minutes and two hours, depending on the urgency. If there is no improvement use conventional medicine unless it is safe to try another homeopathic remedy. If the treatment is helping, wait. If the condition then gets worse again, or stops getting better, more tablets should be given.

3: MILD ACUTE ILLNESSES

These are illnesses such as colds, flu, mild infections and injuries and a whole host of common ailments.

Professional Help: This is not essential as long as the condition does not deteriorate. In this category it is safe for you to give homeopathic treatment while monitoring the patient. Some of these illnesses will

LEFT MILD COMPLAINTS, WHICH INCLUDE THE COMMON COLD, CAN BE
TREATED WITHOUT PROFESSIONAL HELP.

be too mild to need treatment, and should be left to take their natural course.

Dose: One tablet of low potency every two hours for four doses. A single dose of potency 30 or higher.

Assessment: Wait for 3–24 hours depending on the severity and pace of the illness. Illnesses such as flu where the onset has been gradual may not respond to homeopathy until the following day. On the other hand, a child with earache in this category should start to get better after a few hours. If there is no change after these waiting times give a new remedy. If the patient is starting to improve then wait. Repeat the treatment if the improvement begins to wears off or comes to a halt.

For the use of Homeopathic Remedies in Chronic Illnesses *see* chapter 10, pp.108–109.

53

CASE-TAKING –
THE ACUTE CASE

Case-taking of acute illnesses concentrates on the here and now of the problem. Whether it is a bruise or pneumonia, the present symptoms will guide you to the right remedy. As far as the choice of remedy is concerned, the patient's normal state of health can be ignored.

When you begin, your patient will usually tell you straight away some basic information. Use that as a starting point to map out the entire geography of the case.

THE AIM OF CASE-TAKING

Your aim is to record a complete symptom picture of the patient. A well-taken case conveys the individual nature of a particular illness and patient. A carefully noted case is a patient half cured. From the record you will be able to decide the urgency of the case, what kind of illness is involved, and which remedy is required.

THE METHOD OF CASE-TAKING

Begin by observing and absorbing – soak up information like a sponge. Use all your senses, especially your eyes. Write everything down and take your time. Do not at this point ask any of the questions that may occur to you. Have minimum impact on what you are observing. If you step into a pool, the ripples spoil the reflection. Instead, make a note of lines for further enquiry. Concentrate on noticing as much as possible about the patient and his/her environment. First impressions can be important and can easily be forgotten. The process is patient-centred – put yourself in his or her position and try to share in the patient's experience.

54

RIGHT NOTE-TAKING IS AN IMPORTANT PART OF HOMEOPATHIC PRACTICE. TRY TO GET AS MUCH DETAIL AS POSSIBLE FROM YOUR PATIENT.

Record the patient's own words as these give a sense of his or her inner state. When the patient has finished speaking, ask him or her to tell you more about each of the things that has been said. Write everything down – its significance may only become clear later. Then ask if there is anything else that has not been mentioned. Give the patient time to think – and then give yourself time to think about what else you need to know. The case-taking check list on p.56 gives you an idea of what needs to be covered.

Do not ask these questions directly. Try to be skillful in raising a subject that you want to know more about. That way the patient will volunteer information that is important to him or her and therefore important in the choice of remedy.

Anything that influences a symptom for better or worse is called a *modality*. For example, cold air may make the patient feel worse, whilst a warm drink makes them feel better. Modalities are important in the choice of remedy, so they should always be included in your notes. They tell us the mode of action of the vital energy of the patient. Modalities that apply to the whole patient are called *general modalities* and are especially important.

55

If there is a pain, find out what it feels like and where exactly it is. Find out what makes each symptom better or worse. For example, does movement make the patient feel better or worse? Also, how did the illness start and did something bring it on?

Always ask open questions such as 'Is there anything that makes your throat better or worse?' rather than closed questions such as 'Do hot drinks help?' Closed questions do not give reliable answers, and, moreover, the answers do not tell you about the intensity of that particular symptom.

In your notes underline the things that are most intense or are stated forcefully by the patient. The most intense things can be underlined three times.

If possible, ask the people close to the patient for their observations. This can help to complete the picture and get the patient's account into perspective.

THE CASE-TAKING CHECKLIST

First, observe and listen to your patient, then pursue lines of investigation arising from their comments. Finally, look through this list. But do not go through it mechanically, rather use it to open up new areas of investigation.

Look at the presenting problems. Note all the symptoms the patient has – where each symptom is, how it feels and its modalities.

Is there anything else? Repeat the sequence of enquiry for any other symptoms.

How did the illness begin? Was the illness triggered by something such as getting cold, or by stress? How long did it take to start?

What is the general state of the patient? Thirsty? Hot or cold? Perspiring? Is he or she hypersensitive to anything? How is the patient affected by the time of day or night, the position he or she adopts, rest, movement, activities, cold or hot applications, bathing etc? How does the environment affect him or her. For example temperature, fresh air, draughts, noise, light, smells, food and drinks, the presence of other people, etc? How is the patient's body functioning in terms of restlessness, perspiration, thirst and hunger? Is he or she wanting or disliking certain foods or drinks? How is the patient sleeping? What affects his or her sleep?

What is the patient's psychological state? Get a sense of the patient's mood (e.g. irritable, angry, sad, changeable, etc.) How is the patient behaving – weepy, aggressive, needy or withdrawn? Is the patient bad-tempered, worrying? Does he or she like attention or have fears, anxieties, etc. Is the patient jumpy, nervous, apathetic, confused or behaving strangely?

When you have recorded everything you can go on to the next stage.

RIGHT USE THIS LIST AS A GUIDE TO TAKING NOTES.

ORGANIZING YOUR NOTES

At first your notes may appear chaotic, but homeopathy has a way of introducing order into this apparent chaos. The notes you have taken all record symptoms of one sort or another. Some are more important than others in the choice of remedy. There are three criteria to apply:

THE HIERARCHY OF SYMPTOMS

This is the order of importance of human functions in selection of the remedy.

Psychological symptoms

These concern the patient's emotional and mental state and behaviour, and are most imortant.

General symptoms

These concern the whole person and the patient will say 'I am' or 'I feel'. For example, sweating at night or a desire for cold drinks.

Local symptoms

These are symptoms of one part of the body, for instance stomachache or a chest pain, and are of least importance.

STRANGE SYMPTOMS

Symptoms can be common or unusual symptoms. In a chest infection it is not surprising if the patient has a cough. A cough that is not bringing up any phlegm is a little more unusual. If the cough is relieved when the patient lies down that is surprising and therefore important.

INTENSE SYMPTOMS

Symptoms that are intense or stated emphatically you should underline up to three times.

RIGHT A DESIRE FOR COLD DRINKS IS A GENERAL SYMPTOM.

Now you should make a list of up to about six main symptoms. At the top will be strange psychological symptoms with three underlinings, if there are any. An example would be the patient being convinced he is about to die because he has an earache. The list will continue down the hierarchy with the intense and strange symptoms given priority. If you were to continue right down the list, at the very bottom would be common local symptoms not underlined, such as slight diarrhoea during a tummy upset.

WORKING OUT THE REMEDY

You now have a manageable symptom picture that you can compare with remedy pictures until you find the most similar one. With your necessarily limited knowledge, however, this presents a problem. It would take ages to look through even the small selection of remedies in this book, so a short cut is needed. The ideal solution is provided by homeopathic repertories, which are indexes of all possible symptoms. After each entry there is a list of all the remedies that can cause that symptom in the provings. This does not mean you can give any of those remedies, however. You need to cross-reference until you find a remedy that covers the whole case.

Repertories tend to be huge books. The most popular basic repertory has 1,200 pages and was put together by Dr James Tyler Kent at the turn of the century. Its publication was a landmark in the evolution of homeopathy.

These very desirable works are not often available to beginners. Instead, you can refer to the list of common acute illnesses in chapter 7 (see pp.65–74). This short cut works reasonably well. Each illness is followed by a list of possible remedies. Now you have only to look through a handful of remedy pictures.

Each remedy picture is presented in hierarchical order to make comparison easier. When comparing the symptom picture of the patient with the remedy picture, be flexible and creative. It is unusual to get a case where all the symptoms fit one remedy. Arriving at the correct remedy is like identifying a flower in a botanical book. There always seem to be several possibilities and the decision is complex. First select the remedies that look possible and hopefully there are only about three or four. Rearrange the pieces of the puzzle in your mind until you come up with a combination that matches one remedy clearly.

Your choice of remedy should not be based on any one main symptom. Think holistically – consider all the main symptoms. Clarify in your mind the overall themes of the illness such as weakness in one case or intense heat in another. The case as a whole is a picture with certain essential features. Most of the essential features and the overall character of the symptom picture should match the remedy picture. When you have narrowed the possibilities down to a few remedies, some of the symptoms lower down the list may help with the final choice. Talking to the patient again may also be helpful. Don't forget to ask about the modalities of each symptom and of the whole person. Even if the remedy you choose is not the best one it may help a little, and will do no harm.

Go by the symptoms, not the disease. A homeopathic remedy works by enhancing the vital energy of the patient. The energy of the remedy must correspond to the energy of the patient. To prescribe a remedy you must know the state of that vital energy. This is not visible – it can be understood only by studying the symptoms. This does not, however, mean that homeopathy simply treats the symptoms. This criticism sometimes levelled at homeopathy is based on a misunderstanding. The remedy is chosen according to the symptoms but works on a deeper level.

Homeopathic skill lies in assessing the symptoms in order to understand the message from the vital energy. The name of the remedy required is written in the language of nature, in the symptoms. The remedy needed does not depend on the name of the disease. Remember that you are treating the patient and the patient will then heal the disease.

CASE HISTORY

A friend asks you to help her 12-year-old daughter who has yet another throat infection. You agree to go and see her with your homeopathic remedies and books. You discover that the girl came home from school two days ago feeling hot, with a headache and sore throat. She developed a fever and was really ill the following morning. She has been sitting or lying on the settee, eating nothing and drinking little. She is hot with fever and a little sweaty and flushed. Looking into her mouth you can see that her tonsils are swollen and red – the left being easily visible. She says that her throat hurts a lot. She will drink only cold drinks because hot drinks make her throat worse. You notice that the patient is sitting away from the heater and looks miserable.

You consult the *case-taking checklist* (*see* p.56) to find out what else you may need to know. Having already covered everything except the patient's general state you ask open questions about that. Your friend, in reply to your question about whether her daughter is better or worse at any time of day or night, says that today and yesterday she was noticeably in more pain first thing in the morning. All other lines of enquiry yield nothing, so your case notes are now complete.

Professional Help: These throat infections can linger for over a week. Your friend already has antibiotics after visiting the doctor but is reluctant to give them to her daughter. You decide that this is a mild acute illness and it is safe to try homeopathy.

Main Homeopathic Symptoms: Worse on waking, worse on left side. Throat pain, worse for hot drinks. The other symptoms are not marked or unusual enough to take into account.

Case Analysis: You consult the list of remedies for throat problems. After writing down the list you look up the remedy pictures. You are looking for a remedy that has the two modalities: worse on waking and worse left side. Eventually you discover that *lachesis* covers these two symptoms and covers the general character of the case.

Prescription: You have *lachesis* in the 30th potency so you give one tablet and go home, asking your friend to telephone you after about six hours. This is a suitable waiting time for a slow-paced acute condition.

Assessment: At that time the patient is reading and is more lively. She says her throat still hurts and she still has a fever. You interpret this as a good reaction so far and decide to await further progress. The next day she is fine. The *lachesis* has worked well as an acute remedy.

Comments: Note that many of the characteristic symptoms of *lachesis* are absent, but this does not matter. The important thing is that what is there fits *lachesis.* There are no psychological symptoms of any significance so general symptoms come to the top of the list. There are two of these, and both of them are strongly suggestive of *lachesis.*

The symptoms of importance in choosing the remedy are not the obvious ones, i.e., sore throat and fever. A sore throat or fever can be cured by many remedies. The individual symptoms of the patient tell us which is the correct one.

POTENCY, DOSE AND REPETITION

In homeopathic evening classes, and at the beginning of college courses, teachers are often besieged by questions about potency, dose and repetition. There are so many different recommendations that newcomers to homeopathy are confused before they start. This section gives guidance on this. The basic principles are simple and will soon become clear.

One of the most confusing things you can do is take lots of different homeopathic remedies either at the same time or too soon after one another. The results achieved are at best mediocre. If you are treating yourself, discussing things with a friend who is also interested in homeopathy helps to get things into perspective. Treating friends or members of your family is easier, but demands emotional detachment in order to make the right decisions.

The best procedure is outlined on pp.51–53 and 108–109. To go on to a new remedy too soon will stop the previous one working. The waiting time is different in the four categories. In urgent cases the correct homeopathic remedy will work very quickly, and it is important not to wait too long before giving a new remedy. In chronic cases, however, it is all too easy to make the mistake of not waiting long enough.

RIGHT POTENCY AND REPETITION OF REMEDIES DEPEND ON THE CONDITION TO BE TREATED.

Once improvement has begun, stop the treatment. Repeat the dose later if the condition gets worse again. Remedies repeated in this way at the right time have a cumulative effect. Remember that homeopathy involves small doses. Successful prescribing includes long periods of time where no treatment at all is given. Vital energy likes to be given a boost then left to work out its own solutions. Give the patient a push in the right direction then wait to see how far he or she gets. When the patient is flagging give another. Sooner or later the patient will keep going unaided.

When one potency of a remedy has been helping and then no longer works, change to a higher potency of the same remedy.

ASSESSING THE EFFECTS OF THE TREATMENT

After waiting the required time, record the changes in the condition of the patient. Give particular attention to any changes in the general state of the patient. At this stage the patient may only just be starting to improve. They may appear to be more their usual self, have more energy or be less affected by the illness. Increased discharges, such as coughing up mucus in chest conditions or the appearance of skin

SELECTING THE POTENCY AND DOSE

Stick to the potencies below 30 at first. When you have read this book and had some experience you may want to use potency 30, which requires fewer repetitions. Do not use higher potencies (200, 1,000, 10,000, etc) without further training. The higher potencies can occasionally over-stimulate the vital energy and cause unnecessary aggravations. In skin complaints, stick to the potencies below 30 for the same reason.

eruptions, are also early signs of improvement. If the patient goes to sleep in an acute illness, this is also a sign of improvement. Similarly, in a chronic illness old symptoms may come back. If one or more of these changes is taking place and the patient is not getting worse in other ways, then the remedy is probably working and you should give no more treatment at this point.

You may be in a dilemma here. Is the remedy starting to work, which means it is important not to interfere? Or is the patient not really any better, and in need of a new remedy? It will become clear one way or the other if you follow the guidance in the tables.

In acute illnesses the patient just gets better when given the right remedy – there are no 'aggravations'. These happen only in chronic illnesses where there is a backlog of symptoms and the patient cannot get better without throwing them out. They are severe in only a very small percentage of cases, and sometimes people who know a little about homeopathy anticipate them unnecessarily.

INDEX OF ACUTE ILLNESSES

CHAPTER SEVEN

To use this section, decide what condition or illness you are treating and then find it in the following list. Write down the possible remedies and study each one in the remedy pictures that follow. The remedy that matches the symptom picture of the patient is the one to give.

The remedies listed will cover most cases you treat. Sometimes an illness will appear with an unusual symptom picture that is beyond the scope of this book.

Some remedies are needed more often than others. Those in capital letters are needed most often, those in italics less often and those in ordinary type sometimes. If you are unable to choose between two remedies, give the one that is statistically the most likely. Chronic illnesses have not been included in this list. Homeopathic remedies are normally referred to by an abbreviation of their Latin name, and this convention is used here. For the full name of each remedy, refer to the Remedy Abbreviations chart on pp.119–120.

ABDOMINAL PROBLEMS: *see* Digestive Problems.

ABSCESSES AND BOILS (*see also* Mastitis): *arn.*, ars., *bell.*, *hep. sulph.*, lach., merc., SIL., sulph.

ALLERGIC REACTIONS (see also Hay Fever): ALL. CEP., APIS, ARS., *euphr.*, *nat. mur.*, *nux vom.*, *puls.*

ANAEMIA: *see* Weakness.

APPENDICITIS: bell., BRY., lach., lyc., merc., *phos.*

BACK PROBLEMS AND SCIATICA: *arn.*, *bry.*, *hyper.*, mag. phos., *nux vom.*, *rhus tox.*, ruta, staph.

BEREAVEMENT: *see* Grief.

BLACK EYE: *see* Eye Injuries.

BOILS: *see* Abscesses and Boils.

BIRTH, FOR THE MOTHER, RECOVERY FROM: ARN., bellis, hyper., staph.

BITES AND STINGS: *apis*, arn., *bell.*, *hyper.*, lach., LEDUM, staph., urt. u.

BLEEDING: arn., bell., cal., carbo veg., ferr., ferr. phos., *ham.*, *ipec.*, PHOS.

BLISTERS: *see* Skin Problems or Burns.

BLOOD POISONING: arn., *ars.*, bapt., echin., *lach.*, pyrog.

BREAST FEEDING PROBLEMS: (*see also* Mastitis) Cracked or Sore Nipples: arn., cal., graph., phyt. Excess Milk: bell., bry., puls., urt. u. Insufficient milk: bell., BRY., puls., *urt u.*

BREATHING DIFFICULTIES AND ASTHMA ATTACKS: acon., *ant. tart.*, *apis*, ARS., bry., *carbo veg.*, cham., cina., *ipecac.*, kali carb., lyc., nux vom., *phos.*, *puls.*, samb., spong.

BROKEN BONES: ARN., bry., rhus tox., symph.

BRONCHITIS: *see* Chest Problems.

BRUISES: ARN., *bellis.*, hyp., led., ruta., symph.

BURNS AND SCALDS: ars., cal., CANTH., *caust.*, ham., hep. sulph., hyp., *kali bich.*, phos., *urt. u.*

CATARRH: *see* Chest Problems, Hay Fever.

CHICKEN POX: ANT. TART., apis, *ars.*, *bell.*, merc., *puls.*, RHUS TOX.

CHILBLAINS: cham., *bell.*, petr., puls.

COLDS: normally straightforward common colds should not be treated. If they persist constitutional treatment is needed.

COLIC: *see* Digestive Problems.

COLD SORES: cal., dulc., graph., nat. mur., *rhus tox.*, sep.

COLLAPSE: acon., arn., ars., carbo veg., verat alb.

CONJUNCTIVITIS: *see* Eye Infections and Inflammations.

COUGHS: *see* Chest Problems and Coughs.

67

CHEST PROBLEMS AND COUGHS: (*see also* Allergic Reactions, Breathing Difficulties and Asthma Attacks, Hay Fever): acon., ant. tart., apis., ars., *bell.*, *bry.*, *carbo veg.*, *caust.*, cham., cina, dros., ferr. phos., hep. sulph., ign., *ipec.*, kali carb., lach., *lyc.*, merc., nux vom., PHOS., puls, rhus tox., rumex, sil., spong., sulph.

BARKING COUGH: acon., *bell.*, *dros.*, hep. sulph., spong.

CHOKING COUGH: hep sulph., IPECAC., kali carb., lach.

COUGH, WORSE FOR DEEP BREATHING: acon., bell., *bry.*, hep. sulph., *kali carb.*, lyc., merc., puls., rhus tox., rumex.

COUGH DURING FEVER: acon., ars., *bell.*, bry., IPECAC., *kali carb.*, nat. mur., nux vom., *phos.*, sabad.

COUGH, BETTER FOR RAISING PHLEGM: hep., ipec., lach., phos.

COUGH, WORSE FOR TALKING: bell., caust., *dros.*, hep. sulph., lach., merc., PHOS., rumex., spong.

COUGH WITH RATTLING IN CHEST: ant. tart., bell., bry., *caust.,
ipecac.,* nux vom., puls., sil.

CROUPY COUGH: ACON., ars., *bell.,* cina., *hep. sulph.,* lach., phos.,
rumex., samb., spong.

PAINFUL BREATHING: acon., *bell.,* BRY., carbo veg., *caust.,* dros.,
phos., nux vom.

PAINFUL COUGH: all. cep., BRY., caust., merc., *nux vom.,
phos.,* rhus tox.

CRAMP: bell., cina., *coloc., mag. phos., nux vom.*

CROUP: *see* Coughs, croupy.

CUTS: *see* Wounds.

CYSTITIS, URETHRITIS: ars., apis, bell., CANTH., caust., equis.,
merc., nat. mur., *nux vom.,* puls., SARS., *staph., sulph.*

DEHYDRATION: Carbo veg., CHIN., phos., puls., *staph.*

DENTISTRY, AFTER: ARN., hyp., led., nux vom., ruta.,
phos., staph.

DERMATITIS: *see* Skin Problems.

DIAPER RASH: *see* Nappy Rash.

DIARRHOEA: *see* Digestive Problems.

DIGESTIVE PROBLEMS: ant. tart., ARS., bell., *bry.,* carbo veg.,
cham., coloc., gels., *ipecac.,* kali carb., LYC., mag. phos., *merc.,* nat.
mur., NUX VOM., op., podo., phos., puls., sulph., verat. a.

COLIC: bell., cham., coloc., mag. phos., nux vom., staph.

FROM FOOD POISONING: ars., carbo veg., lach., lyc., merc., puls.

FROM OVERINDULGENCE: ant. c., ars., ipecac., lyc.,
nux vom., sulph.

FROM EMOTIONAL UPSETS OR NERVES: arg. nit., cham., coloc., gels., ign., lyc., puls., op., staph.

FROM TEETHING: ars., bell., CHAM., cina., *rheum.*

TRAVELLER'S TUMMY: ars., lyc., nux vom., puls.

WITH WIND: arg. nit., carbo veg., *lyc.,* nux vom.

WITH CHILL: ars., phos., verat. a.

DISLOCATIONS: arn., bry., rhus tox., ruta.

EAR INFECTIONS AND EARACHES: *acon., bell.,* cham., *ferr. phos.,* hep. sulph., lach., lyc., *merc.,* phos., *puls., sil.*

EMOTIONAL PROBLEMS: (*see also* Grief and Nervousness) The following remedies may also be needed for any illness accompanied by these emotions.

ANGER: CHAM., *coloc., hep.,* ign., NUX VOM., *staph., stram.*

ANXIETY: acon., *arg. nit.,* ARS., bry., caust., *gels.,* lyc., puls.

BEING CRITICAL OR FUSSY: ARS, *NUX VOM.,* VERAT. A.

DISLIKE OF SYMPATHY: ign., *nat. mur., sep.*

EXCITEMENT: coff., gels., ign., phos., puls., staph.

FRIGHT OR FEAR: ACON., *ars.,* bell., ign., op., *phos.,* puls., *stram.*

JEALOUSY: apis, ign., LACH., nux vom., puls., staph.

SADNESS: gels., ign., nat. mur., puls.

WEEPING: apis, ign., PULS.

EYE INFECTIONS AND INFLAMMATIONS: *acon., all. cep., apis,* ars., *bell.,* bry., *euphr.,* lyc., *merc.,* nux vom., *puls., staph.*

EYE INJURIES: *arn., cal.,* euphr., *led.,* staph., SYMPH.

69

EXHAUSTION: ant. tart., bry., carbo veg., gels., merc., nux vom., phos.

FAINTING OR FAINTNESS: carbo veg., op., puls.

FEVER: ACON, apis, *ars.*, BELL, *bry.*, cham., FERR. PHOS., *gels.*, *lyc.*, *merc.*, *nat. mur.*, *nux vom.*, *phos.*, *puls.*, rhus tox.

FLU: acon., ars., bell., *bry.*, *eup. perf.*, *ferr. phos.*, GELS., *nux vom.*, phos., puls., rhus tox.

FOOD POISONING: *see* Digestive Problems.

FOREIGN BODIES: hep. sulph., *sil.*

FRACTURES: *see* Broken Bones.

GASTROENTERITIS: *see* Digestive Problems.

GERMAN MEASLES: acon., BELL., *ferr. phos.*, *puls.*

GOUT: *bell.*, *led.*, puls., *urt. u.*

GRAZES: *see* Wounds.

GRIEF: IGN., nat mur., *puls.*, *staph.*

GUM BOILS: *see* Abscesses and Boils.

HAY FEVER: ALL.CEP., *ars.*, euphr., nat. mur., nux vom., puls., sabad., sil.

HEADACHES AND MIGRAINES: ars., bell., *bry.*, gels., ign., lach., lyc., nat. mur., *nux vom.*, phos., puls.

HEAD INJURIES: ARN., hyp., led.

HEARTBURN: *see* Digestive Problems.

HEAT EXHAUSTION, SUNSTROKE: acon., BELL., bry., gels., *glon.*, lach., nat. mur., puls., verat. a.

HEAT RASH: *see* Skin Problems.

HEPATITIS: ars., bell., bry., *chel.*, LYC., merc., nux vom., phos.

HERPES SIMPLEX: *see* Cold Sores.

HERPES ZOSTER: *see* Shingles.

HIVES: *see* Skin Problems.

HOUSEMAID'S KNEE: *see* Injuries.

IMMUNIZATION, ILL EFFECTS OF: acon., *apis*, ars., *bell.*, merc.

IMPETIGO: ars., graph., merc., rhus tox., sulph.

INFECTIONS: *see* under part of body infected

INFLUENZA: *see* Flu

INJURIES: (*See also* Bites and Stings, Broken Bones, Burns and Scalds, Eye Injuries, Head Injuries, Wounds) ARN., bellis., bry., *cal.*, hyper., *led.*, phos., staph., *symph.*, *rhus tox.*, ruta.

OF JOINTS: bry., *rhus tox.*

HICCOUGHS: ign., mag. phos, nux vom.

HOMESICKNESS: *bry.*, ign., merc., staph.

INSOMNIA: *see* Sleeplessness.

JET LAG: *arn.*, cocc., gels.

JOINT INJURIES: *see* Injuries.

KIDNEY PROBLEMS: APIS, *ars.*, BELL., *berb.*, bry., *canth.*, lyc., puls.

LARYNGITIS: acon., bell., dros., gels., phos., spong.

MALARIA: chin., *nat. mur.*, nux vom.

MASTITIS (AND BREAST ABSCESSES): apis, BELL., BRY, hep., lach., lyc., merc., phos., puls., *phyt.*, sil.

MEASLES: acon., *apis*, *ars.*, BELL., bry., euphr., *ferr. phos.*, gels., *puls.*

MENINGITIS: acon., *apis*, BELL., bry., lach., merc., phos., stram.

MIGRAINES: *see* Headaches and Migraines.

MORNING SICKNESS: *see* Nausea in Pregnancy.

MOTION SICKNESS: *see* Travel Sickness.

MUMPS: acon., apis, ars., *bell.*, bry., cham., lach., lyc., *merc.*, phyt., pilo., *puls.*, rhus tox.

NAILS, INFLAMED OR INFECTED: bell., hep., sil.

NAPPY RASH: apis, ars., *bell.*, cal.

NAUSEA AND VOMITING: *see* Digestive Problems.

IN PREGNANCY: ipecac., kreos., *nux vom.*, *puls.*, *sep.*, tab.

NERVOUSNESS (ANTICIPATION): *Arg. nit.*, *gels.*, lyc.

NOSEBLEEDS: acon., arn., bell., bry., *ferr. phos.*, ham., lach., led., *phos.*

OPERATIONS: *see* Surgery, after.

OVEREXERTION: arn., rhus tox.

PERIOD PAINS: bell., caul., cham., cimic., coloc., lach., mag. phos.

PLEURISY: *see* Chest Problems.

PNEUMONIA: *see* Chest Problems.

PRICKLY HEAT: *see* Skin Problems.

RASHES: *see* Skin Problems.

RETENTION OF URINE: acon., *apis*, arn., ars., bell., *caust.*, op.

RINGWORM: graph., sep., sulph.

RUBELLA: *see* German Measles.

SCALDS: *see* Burns and Scalds.

SCARLET FEVER AND SCARLATINA: apis, BELL., bry., cham., lach., lyc., merc., phos., rhus tox.

SCIATICA: *see* Back Problems.

SCRATCHES: *see* Wounds.

SEPTICAEMIA: *see* Blood Poisoning,

SHINGLES: apis., ARS., hep., lach., merc., RHUS TOX.

SHOCK: acon., ARN., ign., op.

SINUSITIS: *see* Colds.

SKIN PROBLEMS: ars., apis, bell., cham., graph., hep., merc., rhus tox., urt. u.

SLEEPLESSNESS: acon., ars., cham., *coff.*, *ign.*, nux vom., phos.

SPLINTERS: *see* Foreign Bodies.

SPORTS INJURIES: *see* Injuries.

SPRAINS, STRAINS: *see* Injuries.

STINGS: *see* Bites and Stings.

STOMACH UPSETS: *see* Digestive Problems.

STRESS: *see* Emotional Problems.

STYES: apis, graph., lyc., merc., puls., *staph.*

SUFFOCATION: ant. tart., carbo veg., op.

SUNBURN: bell., cal.

SUNSTROKE: *see* Heat Exhaustion.

SURGERY, AFTER: ARN., *bellis.*, cal., *staph.*, *stront.*, *carb.*

TEETHING: acon., bell., CHAM., cina., ign., kreos., puls., rheum.

TENNIS ELBOW: *see* Injuries.

TETANUS: arn., HYP., *led.*

THROAT PROBLEMS: acon., *apis*, ars., BELL., bry., ferr. phos., hep. sulph., ign., LACH., *lyc.*, MERC., nux vom., puls., rhus tox., sil.

THRUSH, ORAL: ANT. TART., *BOR.*, CHAM., MERC.

   GENITAL: *bor.*, merc., nat. mur., sep.

TIREDNESS: *see* Exhaustion.

TONSILLITIS: *see* Throat Problems.

TOOTHACHE: acon., arn., bell., cham., coff., kreos., MERC., nux *vom.*, puls., STAPH.

TRAVEL SICKNESS: arn., cocc., nux vom., petr., sep., tabac.

ULCERS, SKIN: *see* Skin Problems.

   MOUTH: ars., lyc., MERC.

URETHRITIS: *see* Cystitis.

URTICARIA: *see* Skin Problems.

VACCINATION: *see* Immunization.

VOMITING: *see* Digestive Problems.

WEAKNESS: *see* Exhaustion.

WHOOPING COUGH: ars., bell., DROS., ferr. phos., lyc., puls., rumex., spong.

WOUNDS: apis, cal., *hyp.*, led., staph.

X-RAY AND RADIATION EFFECTS: rad. brom., ruta.

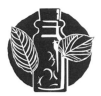

FIRST AID REMEDIES

CHAPTER EIGHT

This section covers all kinds of physical injury, including shock. The remedies used to treat these conditions are those included in the first-aid kit (*see* **pp.44–45**).

ARNICA (the Fall Herb, a mountain flower)
Arnica is an essential first aid remedy. It is needed for many cases of physical injury to any part of the body, from mild bruising to serious trauma and associated shock. *Arnica* may also be needed after dentistry, surgical operations and childbirth if bruising, soreness and possibly shock predominate.

Using *arnica* is an easy introduction to homeopathic prescribing. It is almost a routine prescription for this kind of physical injury – unless the symptoms point to another remedy in this section. Here are some indications for *arnica*:

• Injuries where bruising predominates. For minor bruises that need treatment use *arnica* cream.

• The affected area is usually sore and made worse by touch.

• Patients who are in shock may insist that they are perfectly all right when they are obviously not.

LEFT *ARNICA* CREAM CAN BE APPLIED EXTERNALLY TO BRUISED AREAS.

HOWEVER, IT SHOULD NOT BE APPLIED TO BROKEN SKIN.

• The typical state of shock – confusion, unclear speech, maybe even unconsciousness.

Conditions that can be healed by *arnica* if it is indicated by the symptoms include bruising, sprains, strains, dislocations, broken bones, bleeding (including internal bleeding), nosebleeds, concussion, stroke (cerebrovascular accident), injuries to eyes, teeth and gums, testicular injuries and lingering effects of old injuries.

Do not apply *arnica* cream or lotion to broken skin as it may cause painful inflammation.

If *arnica* is not working well enough in an injury, consider *ruta*, *rhus tox.*, *bellis*, *bryonia*, *ledum* and *symphytum*.

BELLIS (Daisy)

Some cases needing this remedy will be similar to those needing *arnica* – bruising, falls, etc. So if *arnica* is not working, consider *bellis*. In addition, *bellis* has several quite specific uses of its own. It is the first choice for the following:

• Where deeper tissues are affected, such as the abdomen or pelvis, especially after surgical operations.

• Problems that have arisen from getting chilled or wet when hot, (like *rhus tox.*) or eating or drinking something cold.

• Lumps remaining long after an injury.

• Injuries to the breasts.

You may have noticed after cutting the lawn how quickly the daisies flower again. In medicine, as in nature, *bellis* has the power of rapid recovery if the symptoms fit the *bellis* picture.

LEFT THE DAISY, ALSO KNOWN AS THE ENGLISH *ARNICA*, HAS GREAT HEALING POWERS.

BRYONIA (White Bryony, a wild European climbing plant)

Bryonia is the opposite of the *rhus tox.*; everything is nearly always made worse by movement, in some cases even the slightest movement. The patient usually wants to keep perfectly still. Pressure also helps to relieve the pain so the patient may be holding the affected part or lying on it or may like tight bandaging.

The first-aid cases covered by *bryonia* are usually broken bones and sprains. Broken ribs often call for this remedy. Like *rhus tox.*, *bryonia* is a remedy with many uses – a 'polychrest'.

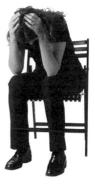

ABOVE PATIENTS TEND TO KEEP COMPLETELY STILL IN A *BRYONIA* STATE AS ANY MOVEMENT MAKES THEM FEEL MUCH WORSE.

CALENDULA (Marigold)

This is the main remedy for skin injuries – grazes, cuts or torn skin. It is excellent as a cream for soothing children's minor skin problems. Larger wounds should be kept completely clean, so do not apply cream or ointment. *Calendula* is also available as a lotion (which should be diluted as instructed on the bottle to prevent stinging) and as tablets. Use the tablets when the injury is more severe, to encourage healing from within, as long as no other remedy is indicated by the symptoms. *Arnica* is usually needed first after a tooth extraction. Give *calendula*, both as tablets and a mouthwash, when bleeding persists.

77

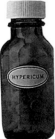

HYPERICUM (St John's Wort)

This herb grows in the wild and in gardens. In homeopathy it is not a treatment for depression. The leaves are full of tiny holes, visible as bright dots when you hold the leaves up to the

ABOVE *HYPERICUM* IS A FIRST AID REMEDY FOR NERVE-RICH TISSUE.

RIGHT ST JOHN'S WORT IS THE SOURCE OF *HYPERICUM.*

light. When you crush the flowers your fingers are left stained red, as if with blood. Here is the *doctrine of signatures* telling us that *hypericum* is good for puncture wounds and bleeding.

• Think of *hypericum* for injuries to parts rich in nerves, such as fingers (tips especially), toes, nail beds, the spine (especially the coccyx, the 'tail bone'), spinal chord and brain, mouth and lips. For example, fingers that have been hit by a hammer or trapped in a door. Also for injuries anywhere that are inordinately painful (showing that nerves are involved) such as nerve pains after dentistry.

• Think of either *hypericum* or *ledum* (*see* below) for puncture wounds where the flesh has been pierced by a nail, splinter or a sting or bite (of plant, insect or animal) or after surgery or injections (especially an epidural). The wound may be inflamed or infected. Pain shooting from the wound up the nerves is a strong pointer to the need for *hypericum*. Successful homeopathic treatment of these wounds automatically helps prevent tetanus or other infections. *Hypericum* may help in tetanus where the wound has affected the nervous system.

ABOVE PUNCTURE WOUNDS RESPOND WELL TO THE *HYPERICUM* REMEDY.

LEDUM (Wild Rosemary)

Use *ledum* first for puncture wounds, bites and stings (as described under *hypericum*) unless another remedy is indicated by the symptoms. This remedy may also be needed for a black eye and occasionally for other dark

RIGHT THE WHOLE WILD ROSEMARY PLANT IS USED TO PREPARE THE *LEDUM* REMEDY.

78

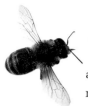

coloured bruises when *arnica* can do no more. The wounded area may feel cold, yet sometimes cold applications help with the pain. *Apis* may also be needed for bites and stings that are relieved by cold applications, but in *apis* the wound feels hot.

ABOVE TREAT BEE
AND WASP STINGS
WITH *LEDUM* IF THE
AFFECTED AREA
FEELS COLD.

RHUS TOXICODENDRON (Poison Ivy)

Rhus tox. is a 'polychrest' – a remedy with many uses. As well as for injuries, it may be needed in throat infections, childhood illnesses, arthritis and many other conditions.

Sprains and strains are the types of injury where *rhus tox.* is most often indicated by the symptoms. The pain or stiffness is nearly always relieved by movement – but getting going is difficult; hence the title 'the rusty gate remedy'. In homeopathic terminology, *beginning to move aggravates, continued motion ameliorates.* A sprained ankle will perhaps hurt most the following morning, or whenever the patient begins to move after being at rest – so he or she may like to keep the joint moving all the time to prevent it seizing up. Sometimes the patient will be so weak or exhausted that he or she cannot move, even though movement would help. Another lead towards *rhus tox.* is an aggravation from getting wet or from damp conditions. Hot bathing, and warmth in any form, help.

Arnica and *rhus tox.* are the two remedies most often called for after overexertion, such as straining to lift something too heavy, or too long in the garden or the gym. (*Arnica* cases are not relieved by continued motion.)

79

RIGHT *RHUS TOX.* IS USED TO TREAT SPORTS INJURIES CAUSED BY OVEREXERTION.

RUTA (Rue, a garden herb)

Ruta is usually required if the injury is sustained in a place where bone is close to the skin. It is the remedy for damage to the surfaces of bones.

Ruta may also be required for sprains and strains, like *arnica*. The injured part may hurt more if lain on, and can feel lame, weak or broken. The pain tends to make the patient restless.

Ruta is often needed for injuries to knees, ankles and wrists, for tennis elbow and for eyestrain (and associated headache). Michelangelo drank rue tea after a hard day's painting.

ABOVE THE GARDEN HERB RUE IS THE SOURCE OF THE REMEDY *RUTA* .

STAPHYSAGRIA (Stavesacre or larkspur, a delphinium)

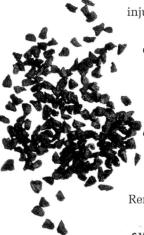

Although occasionally needed for minor skin injuries, stings and bites, this remedy is more often needed for serious injuries or after operations. The wound is hypersensitive, as if the nerves are raw. After an operation the whole body may be reacting as if to an invasion. Any operation could produce this reaction, but especially stretching of body openings and abdominal or pelvic surgery. Information on this remedy will also be found in the Acute Remedy Pictures (*see* p.104).

ABOVE DELPHINIUM SEEDS ARE USED TO MAKE THE REMEDY *STAPHYSAGRIA*. THE REMEDY IS COMMONLY USED BY HOMEOPATHS FOR TREATING POST-SURGICAL WOUNDS.

SYMPHYTUM (Comfrey, or Knitbone)

This is another remedy that has proved invaluable in some specific circumstances. We know from centuries of use as a herb that comfrey can help in many injuries – especially in injuries to bone or cartilage when other remedies are not doing the trick.

- It may be needed in comminuted fractures (when the bone is broken into little pieces) or injuries to hands or feet where small bones, cartilage, tendons and ligaments may all be damaged together.
- For injuries to the eyeball where there is no bleeding.
- For cracked bones, or pain in broken bones that are slow to heal. It will speed up the healing.

ABOVE COMFREY, THE SOURCE OF *SYMPHYTUM.*

LEFT AS ITS POPULAR NAME OF KNITBONE SUGGESTS, COMFREY IS AN EXCELLENT REMEDY FOR BROKEN BONES.

81

TREATMENT FOR BURNS

Various creams and lotions are available for minor burns. They are usually based on a mixture of *calendula, hypericum* and *urtica urens* (stinging nettle). *Urtica* can also be taken as tablets if the pain persists. *Cantharis* (Spanish Fly), taken as tablets, is the usual remedy for more serious burns with blistering or deeper damage, (*see* next chapter). This usually works marvellously to reduce pain, promote healing and help prevent scarring. If the patient is in a state of shock, give *arnica* first, then soon go on to a specific burn medicine. *Causticum* is often required for deep burns that are very painful, and *kali bichromicum* for deeper burns that have penetrated into the tissues, like ulcers. For electrical burns give *phosphorus.* For X-ray burns, sunbed burns, some severe cases of sunburn and for radiation effects generally give *radium bromide.*

REMEDIES FOR COMMON ILLNESSES

This chapter includes remedy pictures that will be useful in treating common *acute* conditions. Each remedy picture describes the illnesses that the remedy can help, together with the physical and psychological state of the patient. The remedy will work if its symptom picture described is similar to the symptom picture of the patient. The whole of the patient must be taken into account to find this similar remedy.

Remember that these remedy pictures are derived from the provings. A large number of people took part in these, and a huge number of symptoms is included. Your patient will have only a few of these and no one symptom is essential. For example, we read in the description of *Aconite: Causation: getting chilled (or, more rarely, overheated), cold wind. Fright, shock, life-threatening ordeals such as mugging, rape, etc. Aconite* could still be the right remedy if the illness was not caused by any of these things. Each patient will only ever have part of the whole symptom picture of the remedy, but the whole of the essential quality of the patient should be there in the remedy picture.

The information is given in the following order – psychological state, general characteristics, modalities, causation, other features etc., illnesses. The similarity between the patient and the remedy in psychological state, general characteristics and modalities is most important. The illness you are treating will usually appear in the list at the end but if not, that does not matter. This is a crucial difference between homeopathy and orthodox medicine. Using homeopathic medicines involves looking at disease in a radically new way.

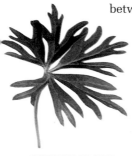

ABOVE: THE LEAVES OF THE
TOXIC *ACONITE* PLANT.

ACONITE (Monk's Hood, *Aconitum Napellus*)
I have been called many times by distressed parents because a child has developed earache, croup, fever or another acute illness suddenly in the night. *Aconite* is often the remedy if the child got cold the previous day.

Psychological State: Fearful – even believing death is imminent. The condition can seem life-threatening to the patient. Sudden frightening illnesses.

General Characteristics: *Aconite* complaints tend to come on suddenly, and be intense. The patient is usually tense, restless and sensitive. There may be tossing and turning. The pain or the illness seem unbearable, the patient demands urgent relief.

Modalities: Worse at night, from dry cold wind, jarring, noise, music, touch and lying on the affected side. Better from perspiration, uncovering and open air.

Other Features: Burning fever, possibly with phases of coldness or paleness. Face alternately red and pale. One cheek red. Dry, barking or croupy cough. Dry eyes, mouth, etc. Intense thirst. Frantic agitation. Violent palpitations. Newborn babies in a state of shock, or with urine retention.

Causation: Getting chilled (or, more rarely, overheated), cold wind. Fright, shock, life-threatening ordeals such as mugging and rape.

83

RIGHT: THE SYMPTOM PICTURE OF *ACONITE*

MAY INCLUDE EARACHE.

Illnesses: Shock, fevers, coughs, croup, earache, asthma attacks, breathlessness, infections, fevers, childhood illnesses.

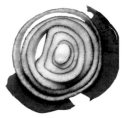

ALLIUM CEPA (Red Onion)

Allium cepa is a constituent of many combination remedies used for hay fever. Everyone knows what onions can cause and cure – watery eyes.

General Characteristics: Inflammations with lots of watery discharges. Burning or smarting pains.

Modalities: Worse in warm rooms. Better in the open air, in cool rooms.

ABOVE: THE COMMON RED ONION IS USED TO MAKE THE *ALLIUM* REMEDY.

Other Features: The nasal discharge burns, but the tears do not (the reverse of *euphrasia*). Coughing and sneezing together. One nostril runny. Colds in damp weather.

Illnesses: Allergies, hay fever, eye inflammations and coughs.

84

ANTIMONIUM TARTARICUM (Antimony potassium tartrate)

Ant. tart. is made from black antimony, which sinks to the bottom of the container when it is prepared chemically and sticks there. It gets its name from Tartarus, the mythological lowest region of the underworld, from which it is almost impossible to rise. Part of the symptom picture is of mucus flooding the lungs, which cannot be coughed up.

General Characteristics: Drowsiness, sinking strength. Respiratory and digestive complaints together. Clammy sweat – the face may be pale and sunken; the lips may be going blue.

Modalities: Better in an upright position, after raising mucus. Worse from warmth, milk and when given attention.

Respiratory Problems: The cough is unproductive so the chest is rattling with mucus,

LEFT ANTIMONY, WHICH IS EXTREMELY TOXIC, IS THE SOURCE OF THE REMEDY *ANT. TART.*

causing difficulty in breathing. Vomiting of mucus. Asphyxia of newborn babies. Suffocation, drowning and choking.

Digestive Problems: Nausea that comes and goes. Indigestion from milk in children. Babies with feeding problems and angry crying. Forcible vomiting, or ineffectual efforts to vomit.

Other Features: Complaints of children and the elderly. Some cases of chicken pox, including ones where the rash is not appearing properly.

Illnesses: Respiratory problems, stomach upsets, chicken pox.

APIS (the Honey Bee, *Apis Mellifica*)

This remedy is made from the honey bee. Bee stings cause swelling and burning pains, which gives hints to the use of the remedy. Further insights come from the behaviour of bees – their busy lives, their aggressive reaction to interference and their jealous guarding of the queen. The hives have a special cooling system to prevent overheating.

ABOVE THE HONEY BEE IS THE SOURCE OF THE *APIS* REMEDY.

Psychological State: Sad, weepy, disappointed. Jealous. A 'queen bee' state of mind; touchy, fussy and demanding. Clumsiness, especially dropping things.

General Characteristics: Puffy swellings, sometimes like sacks of water; tight, itchy, painful or red swellings often near the eyes or of the face or throat. Burning or stinging pains. Sudden pains making the patient cry out. Complaints are often worse on, or start on, the right side.

Modalities: Worse after sleep, from touch, from heat in any form. Worse 3–5pm. Better from cold applications, cold drinks, cold air, open windows.

Causation: Emotions such as jealousy and anger.

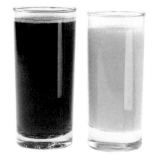

RIGHT THE *APIS* PICTURE IS CHARACTERIZED BY A DESIRE FOR COLD DRINKS.

85

Fever: High fever without thirst, with sleepiness, with sensitive skin. One part hot, another part cold.

Respiratory Problems: When caused by overheating, or accompanied by heat or chill or constricted throat. Panting, gasping for breath, needing the windows open.

Other Features: Symptoms that resemble the effects of a bee sting. Meningitis – the shrieking in the *apis* symptom picture caused by the pain, or coming during sleep or unconsciousness, is like the 'brain cry' of meningitis. Hydrocephalus. Scanty urine.

Illnesses: Allergic reactions, inflammations and infections of any part of the body (including joints and kidneys), respiratory conditions, fever, swellings, oedema, serious effusion, hives, measles, cystitis and any illness where the symptoms indicate apis.

ARSENICUM ALBUM (White Arsenic, Arsenic trioxide)

There is more on the *Arsenicum album* remedy in the case study in chapter one (*see* p.13).

Psychological State: The *arsenicum* patient is typically anxious, restless, critical and fastidious. He or she tends to be a difficult patient – hard to please and intolerant of disorder or mess. He or she is often worried about the illness and fears the worst, needing company and lots of reassurance. The restlessness makes the patient toss and turn in bed, or move around the house, even to try different beds. Fast movement can have a calming effect.

General Characteristics: The patient is usually cold, restless and anxious. Burning pains, but the patient still loves heat. Burning discharges (for example causing sore nostrils in colds and sore anus in diarrhoea). Dryness of the mouth with thirst for frequent sips of liquid (although the patient can also be thirsty for larger amounts). Exhaustion. Illnesses producing sudden or extreme weakness.

Modalities: Worse from about midnight to 2am, from cold, from exertion, from sight or smell of food. Better from warm food or drink and from cool air to the head.

Causation: Food poisoning, cold food, getting chilled, insecurity.

Fever: With great sensitivity to cold. With the feeling of heat internally and cold externally, or vice versa. Burning (or icy coldness) in the blood vessels.

Digestion: Diarrhoea that can be offensive smelling, burning and exhausting. Vomiting. The vomiting can be frequent and very easily induced, e.g. straight after drinking, possibly even the smallest amount (*phosphorus* also has this symptom), on moving, during perspiration.

Other Features: Blackness; of skin, lips, of vomited material etc. Corpse-like body odour. Pale face, haggard expression. Asthma attacks where the patient cannot bear to stay in bed.

ABOVE *ARS. ALB.* PATIENTS FEEL BETTER FOR TAKING WARM DRINKS.

Illnesses: Anxiety states, diarrhoea, stomach upsets, food poisoning, all sorts of infections, inflammations and fevers, common colds, any condition presenting the symptom picture of *arsenicum*.

BELLADONNA (Deadly Nightshade)

My first experience of the dramatic speed with which *belladonna* can sometimes work was one night when my daughter woke up suddenly with a high fever. She was very hot, and obviously having hallucinations. She had gone to bed in a cold room with wet hair.

Psychological State: May be listless, for example during a fever. Can also have hypersensitive senses, or be wild and delirious – behaving violently, muttering or seeing monsters, frightening faces, etc. Frightful nightmares.

General Characteristics: Sudden violent conditions. Heat, bright redness and throbbing of the whole patient or the affected part. Complaints accompanied by shiny or staring eyes, dilated pupils, or flushed face. The patient may radiate heat. A desire for lemonade or lemon juice. Muscular spasms from cramps and twitches to febrile convulsions (convulsions brought on by high fever).

Modalities: Worse at 3pm, on the right side of the body (e.g. earache),

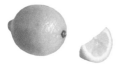

from light, noise and jar; also from allowing the affected part to hang downwards or from lying on the painful side. Better lying on the abdomen or bending backwards.

Fever: With photophobia, with hot head and cold hands and feet. With delirium or hallucinations. With sweat on covered parts.

Other Features: Sensitive head. Congestion of the head. Full hard pulse. Jerking in sleep. May be the remedy for any infections from cystitis to earache (including chest and throat infections).

Illnesses: Fevers, inflammations and infections of all kinds; childhood illnesses, coughs, delirious fevers, headaches, sunstroke, photophobia, abdominal cramps, colic, muscular spasms, inflamed boils, nappy rash, sunburn and all complaints where the symptom picture of *belladonna* is present.

88

BRYONIA (White Bryony, Wild Hops)

Children can throw up very high fevers (for which, incidentally, *belladonna* is often the indicated remedy). It is a sign of their high levels of vital energy and their powerful immune response. The second fever that my daughter had did not call for *belladonna*. She was very, very thirsty, and was delirious, saying 'I want to go home'.

This strange psychological symptom of wanting to go home, even though she already was at home, suggested the remedy *bryonia*. Her great thirst confirmed this.

Psychological State: *Bryonia* patients tend to want to be left alone rather than be fussed over. They can be irritable, for instance, if asked questions. They want stillness of

LEFT *BRYONIA* PATIENTS WANT TO BE LEFT ALONE AND CAN BE EXTREMELY IRRITABLE IF DISTURBED.

mind as well as of body and do not want to think or respond. Usually not talkative, they can however be worried about business or financial matters and talk about them. This applies when they are delirious and they can be obsessed with getting back to work or to their studies.

General Characteristics: There are two important themes in *bryonia* cases – aggravation of the condition from any movement, and dryness (of mucus membranes, lips, mouth, etc). Even the slightest motion may be painful, for example moving the eyes during a headache. In back problems the patient will keep every part of his body still. In chest problems coughing, and even breathing, can be painful.

Other remedies can have this sensitivity to motion (though usually not so intensely), so try to confirm the choice of *bryonia* with other symptoms; thirst for large amounts of liquid, often drunk all in one go; sticking or stitching pains.

Modalities: Worse from motion, warm rooms, warmth generally, in the evening, especially at 9pm, after eating. Better from pressure applied to the painful part, holding the chest when coughing, lying on the painful side, keeping still.

Causation: Financial worries, exposure to cold.

Other Features: Constipation with large dry stool. Constipation on holiday. Digestive problems during fevers or relieved by warm drinks. Gradual onset of illness (unlike *belladonna*). Fever with changeable sequence of heat, chill and sweat, perhaps occurring in the autumn. Increased perspiration in the open air.

Illnesses: May be the remedy indicated in a wide range of illnesses similar to *belladonna*. Dry pleurisy, mastitis, appendicitis, influenza., muscle, back and joint problems.

CANTHARIS (Spanish Fly)
This remedy is used mainly for urinary infections and burns (*see* p.81).
Psychological State: Restless and frenzied due to pain.
General Characteristics: Burning pains. Thirst with no desire to actually drink.

Modalities: Cold applications relieve. Coffee aggravates.

Cystitis: Urgent frequent desire to urinate. Burning pains before, during or after urination, but most often near the beginning.

Illnesses: Cystitis, urethritis, kidney problems, burns.

CARBO VEGETABILIS (Charcoal)

Charcoal is made by burning wood without air. The patient also feels deprived of air, having a hunger for cold fresh air. In charcoal production impurities are driven off in the smoke. The patient also produces noxious fumes, from both ends.

Psychological State: The patient can be unmotivated and not care about his or her state.

General Characteristics: Weak and cold, with cold sweat – yet a strong desire for cold air. Sometimes the patient wants to be fanned. Cold breath, cold tongue. Weak pulse. Pale or blue face and skin. Sluggish weakness, overrelaxation – of the whole person or of lungs or circulation. Feeling full and heavy. Difficulty in breathing. This remedy could be needed in a prolonged illness or a sudden collapse.

Modalities: Better from air (cold and fresh); fanning; passing wind. Worse from exertion, fatty or rich food, in the evening.

Causation: Shock, poisoning (especially by gases), accident, injury, bleeding.

Indigestion: After overindulgence. Fullness and bloating with unpleasant belching or flatulence. Headache with indigestion.

Other Features: Slow bleeding of dark (venous) blood. Puffy, purplish swollen tissue.

Illnesses: Indigestion, collapse, bleeding, breathing problems, coughs, slow recovery from illness or surgery.

ABOVE CHARCOAL, THE
SOURCE OF THE REMEDY
CARBO. VEG.

CAUSTICUM

This mineral compound was created by Hahnemann from slaked lime and potash. It is unknown outside homeopathy.

Psychological State: Tired and weak. Crying easily.

General Characteristics: Trembling, weakness or paralysed feeling.

Modalities: Worse from cold or dry air. Better from cold drinks, cold applications.

Cough: The patient cannot cough up the mucus, or involuntarily swallows it down again. Coughing or sneezing may cause incontinence. Cough relieved by sips of water. Hoarse or weak voice. The chest feels raw and sore.

Face: Neuralgia or paralysis after getting cold, usually on the right side.

Other Features: Frequent swallowing. Burning pains. Burns – severe or chemical, often with blisters. (Slaked lime burns the skin.)

Illnesses: Coughs, paralysis (e.g. of bladder, facial muscles), loss of voice, cramps, burns.

CHAMOMILLA (German Chamomile)

Chamomilla is the well-known saviour of many teething or colicky babies and their parents, except when it does not work and *cina, nux vom., coloc., rheum,* or another remedy is needed. *Chamomilla* is overused because of its reputation. If it is given every time a baby is distressed, the remedy loses its effectiveness.

Psychological State: Irritable, excitable, whining, impossible to placate. Great sensitivity to pain. Pain causes anger. Demanding something then rejecting it.

General Characteristics: Unbearable pains. Sweating or fainting from pain. Pain with numbness. Distressed infants or babies who are whinging or crying frantically, often during teething or colic and need to be carried all the time. Sleeplessness from pain.

Modalities: Worse from attention, touch, being out in wind, warmth, night-time, 9am or 9pm. Better from being carried.

Causation: Teething. Anger. Drinking coffee.

Other Features: One red cheek. Sour body odour.

ABOVE *CHAMOMILLA* IS DERIVED FROM THE GERMAN CHAMOMILE.

Green diarrhoea, perhaps smelling of rotten eggs. Diarrhoea in teething babies. Labour pains sometimes need *chamomilla*. Toothache after getting angry.

Illnesses: Teething, stomach upsets, colic, diarrhoea, ear problems, fevers, sleeplessness.

CINA (Wormseed)

This remedy will cure fevers, coughs and digestive problems if they are associated with the touchy emotional state of *cina*. The patient is usually a child who gets angry at any interference, even if given loving attention.

COFFEA (Coffee)

Coffea cures states of overexcitement, mental hyper-activity, and acute senses. It is often used for sleeplessness. It also covers toothache if the pain responds well to cold water held near the tooth.

ABOVE THE BERRIES OF THE COFFEE TREE ARE THE SOURCE OF THE *COFFEA REMEDY*.

COLOCYNTH (Bitter Cucumber)

The main feature of this remedy is cramping abdominal pains, which make the patient double up. The pains may be relieved by leaning over something hard or by pressing on the abdomen. If *coloc.* is the remedy for colic, then anger is usually the trigger of the problem, or at least the patient is very irritable because of the pain.

DROSERA (Sundew, a carnivorous plant)

This remedy is used for whooping cough or other violent coughs with retching or gagging. The cough may be accompanied by a tickle in the throat, nosebleeds or blueness of the face, and the hours after midnight are the worst time.

LEFT THE CARNIVOROUS SUNDEW PLANT.

EUPATORIUM PERFOLIATUM (Boneset)

The American pioneers used this remedy for 'breakbone fever'. If flu is accompanied by pains in the bones (possibly feeling as if the bones are broken) then *eup. perf.* may be the remedy. There can be a desire for ice-cold water, and early morning tends to be the worst time.

EUPHRASIA (Eyebright)

According to the *doctrine of signatures* the medicinal uses of a plant can be observed in its appearance and habits. Eyebright flowers have purple and yellow spots that resemble bloodshot or diseased eyes. It is used when eye symptoms predominate in such conditions as hay fever, measles and allergic reactions.

The tears or discharges from the eyes are burning to the skin; the nasal discharge is bland. Mucus membranes of the eyes, nose or mouth can be swollen, red and discharging.

93

FERRUM PHOSPHORICUM (Iron Phosphate)

Ferrum phos. is sometimes needed in fevers, infections and inflammatory illnesses that do not have the intensity of *aconite* or *belladonna*. In fact this remedy should be considered in illnesses of that kind that do not seem to fit any other remedy very clearly.

Psychological State: Usually tired and indifferent, but possibly quite alert even when ill; sometimes even cheerful and lively.

General Characteristics: Gradual onset. Blood-streaked discharges, or easy bleeding (e.g., from nose, gums) during fevers etc. Throbbing.

Modalities: Better from gentle movement. Worse on right side from touch, jar, exertion, standing, and at 4–6am.

Other Features: Pale, but possibly flushing easily. Clearly defined red cheeks. Pale mucus membranes. Hard dry tickling cough with sore throat. May be needed after *arnica* in injuries involving bleeding or bruising. Earaches that *belladonna* does not cure.

Illnesses: Coughs and colds, earaches and all kinds of infections, bleeding.

GELSEMIUM (Yellow Jasmine)

This remedy is indicated in some cases of flu. Like *chamomilla*, it is probably used too frequently – make sure the symptoms fit the remedy picture.

Psychological State: Nervous, perhaps trembling. Nervous about forthcoming events such as exams, dental appointments or any ordeal. Tired, dull, heavy, slow, weak and sleepy. Mental paralysis from fear. Blankness of mind.

General Characteristics: Lack of thirst. Weakness: droopy eyelids or jaw. Limbs feel heavy, head needs support. Sleepy look. Weak muscles. Trembling and shivering, worse from exertion.

Modalities: Worse from bad news or excitement. Better from alcoholic drinks, conversation, and after urinating.

Causation: Warm weather after the winter. Flu in spring or autumn.

Other Features: Chills up and down the back, aches all over.

Illnesses: Mainly flu and anticipatory nervousness, but also measles, labour, headaches and diarrhoea.

HAMAMELIS (Witch Hazel)

Hamamelis can give temporary relief for complaints connected with the blood of veins, e.g. varicose veins, piles and bleeding from veins, especially in pregnancy. The affected parts are usually inflamed, sore and made worse by touch. It may be needed for nosebleeds where there is a little bleeding that will not stop, for bruising that persists after *arnica* and to apply to minor burns and wounds.

HEPAR SULPHURIS

Psychological State: Irritability arising from oversensitivity. Oversensitivity to the slightest cold, touch, pain, frustration, etc. The patient tends to be very touchy, dissatisfied and unreasonable. Fainting from pain.

General Characteristics: There is often pus involved in *hepar sulph.* – in throat or skin infections, gum abscesses, etc. The pus may have a bad smell. The affected part is often very sensitive to cold, draughts, touch etc. Pains as if from a splinter or fish bone.

Modalities: Worse from cold, draughts, any part of the body being uncovered, touch. Better from warmth, hot drinks, damp warmth.

Other Features: Needed sometimes for coughs. Croup or croupy coughs worse in cold air. Cough with hoarseness and choking, perhaps with thick yellow mucus.

Illnesses: Coughs and all kinds of infections, usually with the formation of pus.

IGNATIA (St Ignatius' Bean)

Always consider this remedy when someone is devastated by loss or other emotion.

Psychological State: Grief from a death or a relationship break up. The patient may be overcome by feelings or try to control them, but burst into sobs, or laugh then cry, or sigh frequently. Self-blame. Dislike of sympathy. Self-absorption. Changeable moods.

General Characteristics: Changeable symptoms. Fainting or sleeplessness from emotions. The feeling of a lump in the throat. There can be contradictory or surprising symptoms – an empty feeling in the stomach not relieved by eating, indigestion better from eating rich foods, cough worse once the patient starts to cough etc.

Modalities: Worse from tobacco, coffee, strong smells. Better from deep breathing, swallowing. Eating can make the patient better or worse.

Causation: Grief, disappointment, fright, humiliation, being told off, worry, anger.

Other Features: Redness of one cheek. Trembling, cramps. Yawning. Nervous twitches. Tightness between chest and abdomen.

Illnesses: Usually, but not always, emotional states or illnesses brought on by emotions.

IPECACUANHA

This is a South American shrub; the word means 'the roadside plant that makes you sick'.

General Characteristics: Mainly a remedy for coughs and stomach upsets. Nausea or breathlessness accompanying any of the complaints mentioned below.

Modalities: Worse from warmth.

Causation: Punishment, too much rich food.

Other Features: Cough or asthma etc with gasping for air, choking, fast breathing, retching. Whooping cough. Constant nausea, nausea not relieved by vomiting. Bleeding, e.g. of nose or uterus: perhaps foamy or in flushes. Cold sweat of face. Profuse saliva.

Illnesses: Asthma, bleeding, coughs, digestive problems.

KALI CARBONICUM (Potash)

As an acute remedy this is required mainly for back and chest problems. All problems tend to be worse around 3am and better leaning forwards when sitting or kneeling. The back problems typically involve a feeling of weakness in the small of the back or the sensation that the back is broken, and can come on during childbirth.

LACHESIS (Venom of the Bushmaster snake)

This is a fascinating medicine because characteristics of snakes appear in the symptom picture. In snakes the organs of the right side have disappeared to make the body long and thin; the provings of *lachesis* produce symptoms on the left side. Also in the symptom picture is sensitivity of the throat to any constriction – the snake's weak point is its throat, and it stretches to swallow things whole.

Psychological State: The patient can be very talkative, mistrustful or jealous.

General Characteristics: Complaints above the waist are worse on the left side, or start on the left and go to the right. Everything tends to be worse as the patient falls asleep, or on waking.

Modalities: Worse from tight collars (and tight waistbands), warmth.

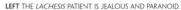

LEFT THE *LACHESIS* PATIENT IS JEALOUS AND PARANOID.

Causation: Jealousy.

Other Features: Blueness or purpleness of affected parts. Sensation of a lump in the throat. Constriction in the throat. Swallowing is painful. Flushes of heat come up the body. Wounds that are slow to heal and turn blue.

Illnesses: Infections of the throat and ear, mumps, septicaemia, bleeding (of dark blood), inflamed wounds, bites and stings, food poisoning.

LYCOPODIUM (Club Moss)

This remedy can be needed in many different illnesses that have the two important modalities of worse at 4pm and worse on the right side.

Psychological State: Nervousness about forthcoming events or new tasks. Lack of self-confidence. A desire for company nearby but not in the same room.

General Characteristics: Desire for hot drinks, which may relieve the symptoms or make the person feel better (but sometimes the patient desires cold drinks). Hunger, with fullness after only a little food. Often indicated in digestive or liver problems where there is bloating and flatulence. Complaints that start on the right side and spread to the left.

Modalities: Worse at 4pm (or 4–8pm), on the right side, from tight clothes. Better after midnight, from passing wind.

Other Features: Yellowness of skin.

Illnesses: Infections (e.g. of ear, throat or chest), digestive problems, liver problems, anticipatory fears, any illness where the symptoms indicate *lycopodium*.

97

MAGNESIA PHOSPHORICA
(Magnesium Phosphate)

A remedy for nerves and muscles, therefore often indicated in conditions such as cramps, spasms, colic and nerve pains. Heat and warm applications such as hot water bottles give relief. The pains can be sudden and violent and shoot around. Pressure on the painful place helps. This pattern could be present in period pains, sciatica, repetitive strain injury (including from playing musical instruments), toothache, etc.

MERCURIUS (Mercury)

Mercury was used widely as a conventional medicine at the time when Hahnemann developed homeopathy. It was a severe treatment, often given until the patient could no longer bear the side-effects, which included profuse salivation, ulcers and purging.

ABOVE STOMACH CRAMPS ARE COMMON IN THE *MAG. PHOS.* TYPE.

Psychological State: Weak and agitated, perhaps hurried. Rapid talking or stammering. Unpredictable behaviour.

General Characteristics: The mercury patient is sensitive to temperature (like thermometers, which make use of this property of mercury), and is usually either too hot or too cold. Nothing seems to help except moderate temperature and rest. Complaints accompanied by excess salivation causing dribbling or dampening of the pillow. Bloody or septic discharges that may burn the skin. Offensive sweat.

Modalities: Worse from both heat and cold, at night, from perspiring.

RIGHT QUICKSILVER, THE SOURCE OF *MERCURIUS.*

Other Features: The mouth is often affected when mercury is needed – the tongue may be flabby and shaped at the sides by the teeth. Also possible are swollen gums, bad breath and a metallic taste in the mouth. Painful diarrhoea.

Illnesses: All kinds of infections including tonsillitis and conjunctivitis, earaches, chicken pox, mumps, swollen glands, diarrhoea, food poisoning, toothache.

NATRUM MURIATICUM

Potentized sodium chloride (common salt) is a more important remedy than its humble origin suggests. It is most often needed as a constitutional remedy, but heals some allergic reactions, catarrhal problems and cases of sunstroke or heat exhaustion.

Salt controls the body's fluids. In the symptom picture there may be dryness, for instance of the eyes, or the other extreme – streaming discharges that are watery or like egg-white. The patient is usually very thirsty, and may get worse at 10am each morning. A special feature of *nat. mur.* is a 'mapped' tongue, where patches of the tongue are discoloured.

NUX VOMICA (Poison Nut)

This remedy is needed for all sorts of conditions.

Psychological State: A *nux vom.* patient tends to be bad-tempered, impatient, critical and hyper-sensitive. This may arise from an inner frustration with hindrances. The senses are acute and noise, smells, pain and discomfort, etc, can annoy the patient tremendously.

RIGHT THE POISON NUT TREE IS THE SOURCE OF *NUX VOMICA*.

General Characteristics: Counter-productive efforts of body or mind, for example constipation with lots of straining, or dogged efforts to achieve misguided aims. Easily chilled.

Modalities: Worse at 3 or 4am and from cold, uncovering, or tight waistbands.

Causation: Overwork. Loss of sleep. Overindulgence in food, alcohol, coffee, drugs or medicines. Getting angry.

Other Features: Sleeplessness from overwork. Cramps, twitching and spasms, muscle spasms, violent vomiting, abdominal cramping pains, spasmodic cough, muscle strains from coughing or sneezing, hiccoughs, sneezing etc.

Illnesses: Back pain, sciatica, digestive problems of all kinds, coughs, asthma, fevers, hay fever, allergies, cystitis, hangovers, travel sickness and any illness that fits the *nux vom.* picture.

OPIUM (Opium Poppy)

Morphine is made from opium and is named after the ancient Greek god of sleep, Morpheus. In material doses it suppresses pain and has a sedative effect, in smaller doses it produces dreaminess and detachment from the world.

In acute homeopathic treatment, *opium* is used to cure those states, whether due to a stroke, a general anaesthetic, a fright or shock, or fever. The patient is usually apathetic, with dulled senses and reduced vital activity (resulting in constipation, weak breathing, etc). There may be a glassy look in the eyes and dark red colouring of the face. High fevers that cause a state of stupor, possibly with snoring.

LEFT APATHY IS ONE OF THE MAJOR SYMPTOMS OF THE *OPIUM* PICTURE.

PETROLEUM (Crude Oil)

This is used as a remedy for travel sickness of car, train, boat or plane when there is also dizziness or headache. Fresh air tends to make the sickness worse.

PHOSPHORUS

This element bursts into flame as soon as it is exposed to the air, and glows in the dark.

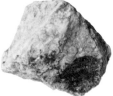

ABOVE THE MINERAL *PHOSPHORUS* IS FOUND IN ALL LIVING MATTER.

Psychological State: Alert and excitable, or burnt out and exhausted. Impressionable, imaginative and fearful of the dark, of being alone and about their illness etc.

General Characteristics: Acute senses. Over-heated from excitement. Burning pains, e.g. in chest or digestive system. Desire for cold food or ice-cold drinks, but sometimes all food and drink are soon vomited. Blood-streaked vomit, mucus or diarrhoea.

Modalities: Worse from cold, change of temperature, on left side, when lying on left side, when lying on the painful side. Better after eating (the patient may be hungry even during a fever or headache), from massage.

Other Features: Profuse red bleeding, e.g. of nose, or from cuts. Heat located in one part of the body or rising up the back. An important remedy for many chest problems, especially left-sided pneumonia. There may be tightness of the chest and loss of voice.

Illnesses: Bleeding, coughs and chest problems, digestive problems, exhaustion, fever, nosebleeds and any illness presenting *phosphorus* symptoms.

PODOPHYLLUM (May Apple)

This is a remedy for diarrhoea that is worse in the morning, even as early as 4am. There may be gurgling in the abdomen leading to gushing diarrhoea that leaves the patient exhausted. This may be caused by teething or hot summer weather. Stroking the tummy helps. Diarrhoea and constipation may alternate.

101

PULSATILLA (the Pasque Flower, or Wind Flower)
There is a characteristic emotional state in this
remedy. Consider *pulsatilla* in any illness when the
patient is tearful and needs a lot of emotional support.
Psychological State: Uncertain and undecided, easily
influenced and perhaps needing lots of reassurance,
affection or physical contact. Changeable moods. The
patient tends to weep easily. Clingy children.
General Characteristics: Changeable symptoms – pains
may move from place to place or the nature of the
complaint itself may change. Very little thirst,
even though the mouth may be dry.
Modalities: Better from fresh air, sympathy,
gentle movement, after crying. Worse from rich
or fatty food, warmth, stuffy rooms.
Causation: After measles, after getting wet.
Other Features: Fainting from too much heat. Profuse bland catarrh.
Illnesses: This remedy can cure any kind of illness when the
symptoms fit the *pulsatilla* picture.

RIGHT *PULSATILLA* IS
PREPARED FROM THE
PASQUE FLOWER.

RHEUM (Eastern Rhubarb)
The symptom picture of this remedy can be similar to *chamomilla*,
with its diarrhoea during teething, sour smelling discharges and bad
temper. Consider it if *chamomilla* does not work.

RHUS TOXICODENDRON (Poison Ivy)
This restless trailing plant was introduced as a medicine 200 years
ago when someone was accidentally poisoned by it; afterwards a
blistery rash of many years duration disappeared.
Psychological State: Weepy, sad or restless.
General Characteristics: Restlessness, due to the fact that continued
movement gives relief of body or mind. Tossing and turning: no
position is comfortable. The patient may become exhausted and
eventually have to rest. Desire for cold milk or other cold drinks.

Modalities: Worse when at rest, on beginning to move, from overexertion, at night, in the autumn. Better from change of position, continued motion, warmth, a hot bath.

Causation: Exposure to cold and damp (e.g. camping) or getting chilled when hot.

Other Features: Redness of the tip of the tongue. Sprains and strains or exhaustion from lifting heavy things, overwork or too much exercise. Skin conditions with burning blisters or an itchy red rash. Hard swollen glands.

Illnesses: Infections and fevers including chicken pox and mumps, shingles, herpes, nappy rash, flu, sore throats, exhaustion, sprains and strains, stiffness, backache, sciatica.

RUMEX
Yellow dock is a remedy for coughs that are made worse by inhaling cold air.

SARSAPARILLA
Wild liquorice is a remedy for cystitis (or kidney infections) when the pain is worse at the end of urinating, when passing the last few drops. Sometimes the pains make the patient scream.

SEPIA (Ink of the Cuttlefish)
This is mainly a remedy for chronic illness (*see* p.113), but may also be needed in pregnancy, childbirth and acute gynaecological problems. The symptom picture includes nausea from smells, especially of food. There can be pains dragging downwards in the uterus region. The person tends to feel worn out and emotionally unresponsive.

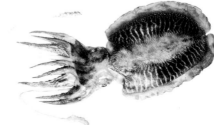

RIGHT *SEPIA* IS PREPARED FROM THE INK
OF THE CUTTLEFISH.

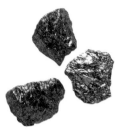

ABOVE *SILICA* IS PREPARED FROM SILICON DIOXIDE, WHICH IS FOUND IN QUARTZ, FLINT AND SANDSTONE.

SILICA

Psychological State: Resignation in the face of stress, fear of failure. Nervousness before important events.

General Characteristics: Cold, tired and weak. Sweat with an unpleasant smell, even when cold, especially on feet, head and the back of the neck. Pains as from a splinter, fish bone, needle, etc. Often given to help expel foreign bodies such as splinters. Fungal infections such as athlete's foot. *Silica* complaints tend to come on slowly.

Modalities: Worse lying on the painful side, after drinking milk.

Causation: Vaccination, or control of a discharge or perspiration.

Other Features: Often needed for septic conditions, boils and abscesses, including those that linger for a long time. Teeth abscesses. The remedy most often needed for babies who vomit breast milk. Lumpy phlegm.

Illnesses: Ear problems, septic conditions, abscesses, some breast-feeding problems, mastitis.

SPONGIA

For some reason powdered burnt sponge came into use as a medicine in the Middle Ages in Europe. In homeopathy, it is used mainly for coughs (usually dry coughs) with breathing difficulties, which may be made worse by exertion, excitement and after sleep. Warm food or drink may help.

STAPHYSAGRIA

(Stavesacre or Larkspur – delphinium)
Needed in many complaints that arise from suppressed emotions, especially unexpressed anger. The person may feel humiliated, invaded or

ABOVE SEA SPONGES HAVE BEEN USED FOR CENTURIES AS A HEALING REMEDY.

104

abused and not be able to do anything about it. Trembling with emotion. Nerves may be hypersensitive.

This remedy is sometimes needed for painful wounds, after surgery (especially if a body opening has been stretched) and in cystitis connected with sexual intercourse.

SULPHUR

Sulphur is one of the most widely used remedies in homeopathy. It is made from flowers of sulphur, a yellow deposit formed by volcanic eruptions. Eruptions, heat and sulphur-like smells are themes in the symptom picture.

Psychological State: Tired, lazy, messy and unconcerned.

General Characteristics: Heat, burning pains, burning discharges. Sore red lips, anus or other body orifices. Flatulence or discharges may smell of rotten eggs. Burning heat of the hands or feet, especially of the soles. A weak, hungry, empty feeling at mid-morning.

Modalities: Worse at 10–12am, from warmth, washing or bathing, while standing.

Other Features: Diarrhoea that forces the patient to get out of bed in the morning.

Illnesses: Any illness presenting the *sulphur* symptom picture.

TABACUM

Tobacco is used to treat some cases of travel sickness, and nausea in pregnancy. With the nausea there may be paleness of the face and sweating. Cool air helps.

URTICA URENS

This remedy has been described in the first aid chapter. It is also required sometimes for hives or prickly heat – and it may regulate the supply of breast milk, when there is too little or too much, if no other remedy is indicated by the symptoms.

RIGHT THE STINGING NETTLE IS THE SOURCE OF *URTICA URENS*.

CONSTITUTIONAL TREATMENT AND DEVELOPING YOUR SKILLS

CHAPTER TEN

In conventional medicine most chronic, or long-term, illnesses are regarded as incurable. The treatment is directed towards controlling the symptoms. Homeopathy, however, has a lot to offer in chronic complaints and can achieve a profound transformation in health.

When you have learnt how to treat acute, or short-term, conditions then you can begin to treat some chronic conditions.

Chronic and constitutional treatment are the same thing. Chronic illnesses arise from the constitution, that is, the psychological and physical type of the patient, and it is this that must be treated. Sometimes constitutional treatment is given when the patient is not particularly ill to prevent illness occurring and to boost general health and well-being.

Much of what you have learned for acute treatment applies to chronic illnesses. A

LEFT WHEN TAKING THE CASE HISTORY OF A PATIENT WITH A CHRONIC COMPLAINT ASK ABOUT HIS OR HER DAILY LIFE.

crucial difference is in the case-taking. The constitutional case-taking extends backwards in time and into the personality and daily life of the patient. Begin by recording all you can discover about the health problems that the patient first mentions. Then ask if there is anything else, letting the patient know that stresses and emotional problems can be included. When you have explored all these issues then check that the following topics have been covered:

ABOVE ANY FOOD AVERSIONS SHOULD BE NOTED IN THE CASE NOTES.

• How the illness (or illnesses) began, and whether any stress or trauma acted as a trigger.

• At some stage in the consultation find out about any difficult phases, stresses or traumas that have affected the patient deeply at any time, from birth onwards.

• Their medical history from birth to the present, including treatments of all kinds.

• Reactions to weather conditions, climate changes, seasons, open air and stuffy rooms, etc.

• Variations in symptoms, energy and mood according to time of day or night.

• General appetite, thirst, food likes and dislikes, and any foods that cause bad effects.

• The quality and pattern of the patient's sleep, including the times of waking and the state of mind; also any recurring dreams.

• For women, any problems associated with the menstrual cycle.

• The emotional characteristics of the person such as anxieties, fears, depression, apathy, nervousness, irritability or anger.

• The patient's responses to other people – family, friends, colleagues and strangers.

• Problems with memory, concentration, understanding, etc.

This list is given to suggest areas for exploration. You can use each item as a starting point and let the patient respond. Follow the patient's lead unless he or she is going off the subject altogether. When a line of enquiry ends, go back to the list.

As always, a homeopath tries to stick to open-ended questions, and to be sensitive to any hints from the patient, conscious or unconscious, of areas that should be explored. Simply asking patients to give a personality sketch of themselves can be very helpful. Record your own impressions of the person.

USING HOMEOPATHIC REMEDIES FOR CHRONIC ILLNESS

Professional Help: Most patients in this category have already been to their doctor, know the diagnosis and may be taking orthodox medicines. You should recommend many of them to see a professional homeopath.

Do not treat any patients who are chronically weak, very elderly or seriously ill. If you decide to treat a chronic skin condition stick to the potencies 6x, 12x and 6c to minimize any aggravation. Remember that oral steroids or antibiotics usually antidote homeopathic treatment.

Dose: One tablet of low potency three times a day for three days, or one dose of potency 30. Always stop the treatment as soon as there is any change in the condition.

Assessment: Assess the effects of the low potencies three days after the treatment is over. Assess potency 30 after 4–6 weeks. With the higher potencies it is sometimes several weeks before the remedy starts to work and patience is needed. If there is no improvement after these waiting times then give a new remedy. If there is an improvement, wait. Repeat the same remedy

LEFT DO NOT TREAT THE VERY ELDERLY FOR CHRONIC COMPLAINTS. THEY SHOULD BE TREATED BY AN EXPERIENCED, PROFESSIONAL HOMEOPATH.

later if the improvement wears off. Patience may be needed here too because, in this category, repeating the medicine at the wrong time or giving a new one can make the treatment ineffective. Do not repeat the treatment for slight or temporary relapses. This is one of the common mistakes in homeopathy.

To work out the remedy *see* pp.58–59. You will also need assistance from some of the books listed in Further Reading (*see* p. 121). Do not give the remedy there and then – think about it for a few days to help get things in perspective.

USING BOOKS

A student of homeopathy studies homeopathic methods and principles, the remedy pictures (*materia medica*) and needs to know how to make good use of a repertory. This is all cemented together by actual experience with patients. This book and the introductory **109** books in the appendix include something of all these and you can begin to treat chronic problems using these introductory books. The advanced books are more specialized and each covers one aspect only. A serious student needs at least three textbooks – a *how-to-do-it* book, a *repertory* and a *materia medica*. The first tells you, among other things, how to use the *repertory* and *materia medica*. After taking the case and putting the symptoms in order, you use the repertory to arrive at a short list of possible remedies. You then study these in the *materia medica* to make the final choice.

To a certain extent the choice of books is a matter of personal preference. However, if you want to put some serious time and study into homeopathy, you will find it hard to

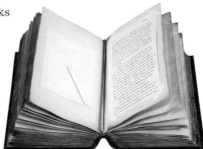

RIGHT *MATERIA MEDICA* BOOKS CONTAIN REMEDY PICTURES AND ARE AN ESSENTIAL TOOL FOR THE SERIOUS HOMEOPATH.

do without *The Science of Homeopathy*, Kent's *Repertory*, or one of the expanded versions of it, and Phatak's *Materia Medica*.

A student must learn about the human body and its diseases. Consider getting a medical text book in addition to a first-aid manual and a family health guide.

FURTHER TRAINING

Try to go to an evening class or an introductory course. If you want to become either a professional homeopath or spend some years studying, details of colleges are available from the professional societies listed at the back of this book (*see* pp.122).

GENERAL GUIDANCE ON CONSTITUTIONAL TREATMENT

When a constitutional treatment is working several things, apart from a straightforward improvement, can happen.

• There can be an aggravation of the symptoms at first.

• The patient may feel better in him or herself before the health problems themselves improve.

• Some of the problems may take longer to get better than others.

• Old symptoms may return briefly.

• A rash or discharge can appear.

To get the best from homeopathy do not give more remedies or other new treatments while these changes are taking place. The temporary return of old symptoms is a good sign and should not be treated. Where there has been a descent into poor health through a series of illnesses, homeopathy can reverse the whole process. The remedy is working holistically, deep within the organism, beyond the level of just one of the diseases. Experiencing homeopathy at work is an education in the true nature of health and disease, and in the nature of the intelligence that the vital energy possesses.

THE LAW OF CURE

Dr Constantine Hering was a homeopath in the United States in the 19th century. His greatest contribution to medicine is called the law of cure and provides a yardstick to assess the overall effectiveness of any kind of treatment. After years of observing patterns of illness in thousands of people over whole lifetimes, Dr Hering saw a progression. If your health is deteriorating, you may find not only that one disease is getting worse, you may also develop new diseases. A common progression in childhood is from eczema to asthma. Conventional medicine also accepts this particular progression. The state of disease has spread from the skin into the respiratory system. Hering's Law tells us that since the lungs are more internal and are more important in the preservation of life than the skin, health in such an event has deteriorated.

This is a statement of Hering's Law – when illness progresses from a less important to a more important organ, or inwards into the organism, then the patient is getting worse, and the treatment is harmful. If the complaints are going in the opposite direction, or in the reverse order of their appearance, then the patient is improving, the treatment is doing good work, and the process must be allowed to continue undisturbed. The body has a natural tendency to cure itself by pushing its problems outwards as discharges or skin eruptions. You can observe this in the childhood illnesses. Many of the worst cases develop if the rash fails to appear properly. These illnesses usually improve once the rash appears. In measles, for example, the virus is killed in the skin rash.

By taking a full medical history, homeopaths track patterns of health carefully. We often see the law of cure operating in our patients – a child's asthma will get better when the eczema he or she had as a toddler reappears. The treatment will then go on to cure the eczema too. Sometimes the same thing happens when treating hyperactivity, and other conditions.

Hippocrates, the father of Western medicine, wrote: 'In those suffering from depression of spirits and kidney disease the appearance of haemorrhoids is a good sign.'

There are very few of these standard patterns of progression. The journey of deterioration and improvement tends to be highly individual, depending on each person's susceptibility (*see* p.24).

These curative reactions are usually mild and trouble free. Homeopaths welcome them because they are followed by long periods of good health. Patients need reassurance that all is well and are usually already feeling better in themselves. It is important not to interfere by giving any new treatment, homeopathic or otherwise, to control these symptoms.

112

CONSTITUTIONAL TYPES

Here are two examples of the dozens of common homeopathic constitutional types.

THE *ARGENTUM NITRICUM* CONSTITUTIONAL TYPE

The *argentum nitricum* remedy is prepared from silver nitrate, a substance used in photographic films because it takes the impression of light and stores the image. The *argent. nit.* type is also impressionable – the kind of thoughts and fears that we can all have briefly and soon forget stay in the mind of the *argentum nitricum* person. This homeopathic type has all kinds of fears and phobias. They can become very nervous before an examination, a visit to the doctor or dentist, any unusual event or anything that seems like an ordeal. Or they may suffer from claustrophobia or agoraphobia. Sometimes, fear and phobias are the result of an overactive imagination. This type can start to imagine all sorts of unlikely possibilities – for example, a person may fear being crushed by a falling building or have a sudden impulse to jump out of the window.

When healthy, this constitutional type is cheerful and extrovert. They love company, are lively and dynamic and rush about a lot. Their excitability and impulsiveness are positive qualities, but can lead to exhaustion.

They are usually warm-blooded people who need fresh air, and often crave salty and sweet foods. The latter can cause bloating and flatulence. Physical problems can be dizziness, catarrh, ulcers, diseases of the nervous system and eye diseases.

THE *SEPIA* CONSTITUTIONAL TYPE

This remedy is made from the ink of the cuttlefish. *Sepia* people are lively and excitable and often love dancing. However, when older or in poor health, their energy level drops both emotionally and physically. They can be undermined by the emotional demands of their family, and may feel drained and unresponsive. The needs of their children and loved ones become a burden to them. They may need to be on their own, dislike sympathy and can be irritable if disturbed.

113

In *sepia* women, the hormonal system can be easily thrown out of balance. There may be all kinds of menstrual and menopausal problems involving vaginal discharges, bearing down pains, prolapses, heavy and prolonged periods, mood changes and exhaustion. *Sepia* is one of the main homeopathic types to suffer ill-effects from pregnancy, childbirth and oral contraceptives.

Two of the personal features that can confirm *sepia* as the right remedy are a desire for pickles or vinegar and a love of dancing and strenuous exercise. Physical exertion seems to lift them out of their lethargy. They may also prefer to keep busy because they feel worse once they stop.

The above two descriptions concentrate on the personality type of the remedies because that is what is most important in selecting constitutional treatment.

CONCLUSION

CHAPTER ELEVEN

Those who have experienced homeopathy working respect and support it. Those who have not are often sceptical and can be totally dismissive. But outright condemnation is decreasing as surveys reveal how widely it is used and how widely its effectiveness is acknowledged. Scientific proof will follow in due course.

Are you now fired by enthusiasm for homeopathy or awed by its complexity? Do you intend to buy all the books and remedies as soon as you can? Or are you uncertain even about taking *arnica* next time you hurt yourself?

After 12 years in full-time practice I am still fascinated by homeopathy and impressed by its power. It is a genuine source of healing. It can amaze people who are new to it, and to dedicated study it gives generous rewards.

This book is quite technical in places. This is necessary because, like any powerful tool, homeopathy must be used properly. And to adjust our way of looking at disease to take on the homeopathic view takes time. In a way, homeopathy turns our notions of health and illness upside down.

Homeopathy is mysterious and yet profoundly practical. Every theory is rooted in observation and every attempt to work out the right remedy receives its acid test when the remedy is given to the patient.

The convenience of keeping and using homeopathic remedies at home means that many households now have some of them, usually *arnica* and a few others. The benefits are not confined to minor ailments. In many cases of serious disease homeopathic remedies offer one of the best chances of real help.

The future for homeopathy looks bright. The approach to health and degree of effectiveness it offers are attracting more and more people, and the demand will continue to increase. Homeopathy has a central role to play in the health revolution that is taking place.

APPENDIX

TESTS SHOWING THE EFFECTIVENESS OF HOMEOPATHY

In the *British Medical Journal* (1943 (ii), page 654) Florey reported that penicillin has effects in dilutions of one part in 250 million (which is like putting one drop of water in 18,000 bottles of whisky!).

In the *Journal of the American Institute of Homeopathy* (1966, no. 59, p.287, and 1968, no. 61, pp.28–9) Anna K Wannamaker shows that homeopathic potencies affected the growth rates of onion seedlings.

Professor Jacques Benveniste's research at the French government research centre INSERM in Paris was published in the scientific journal *Nature* in June 1988. It reported on experiments repeated in three countries that showed that homeopathic dilutions work.

The veterinary surgeon Christopher Day reported in the *British Homeopathic Journal* in January 1986 (no. 75 pp 11–15) that caulophyllum 30c reduced stillbirths in pigs. Christopher Day also featured in a BBC *Horizon* programme, which showed herds of cows getting far less mastitis as a result of homeopathic treatment.

A trial of a homeopathic potency of pollen in treating hay fever proved the remedy six times better than a placebo. (Reilly, Taylor, McSharry and Aitchison; *The Lancet*, 18 October 1986, pp.881–6).

Many more examples are quoted in *Homeopathy: Medicine of the Twenty-First Century* by Dana Ullman (North Atlantic Books, California, 1988) and in *Homeopathic Science and Modern Medicine* by Harris Coulter (North Atlantic Books, California, 1980).

GLOSSARY

>: made better by (for example, sore throat > hot drinks means that the patient's sore throat is relieved by drinking something hot).

<: made worse by. Both symbols are commonly used in homeopathy.

Acute: An acute illness is a short-term illness such as a cold, a digestive upset or pneumonia. An acute illness can be mild or severe.

Aggravation: A temporary worsening of symptoms after taking a homeopathic remedy.

Allopathic Medicine: Orthodox medicine is allopathic, i.e., it uses medicines with effects opposite to the illness.

Antidote: Something that stops homeopathic remedies working. The main examples are coffee, camphor, eucalyptus and menthol.

Case-taking: The recording of all the information about a patient that a homeopath needs.

Centesimal: The scale of potencies that is diluted to one part in a hundred at each stage of **potentization**.

Characteristic Symptoms: Symptoms that are typical of a certain remedy, for example the slow functioning of a *gelsemium* patient.

Chronic: Chronic illnesses are long term illnesses such as eczema and cancer, as opposed to acute illnesses.

Common Symptoms: These symptoms are usually found with a certain disease, for example a cough during a chest infection. They are of little importance in selecting the homeopathic remedy.

Constitutional Treatment: This is treatment of the whole person for long-term health problems.

Conventional Medicine: The mainstream medicine of our times, i.e., **allopathic medicine**.

Decimal: The scale of potencies that are diluted to one part in 10 at each stage of **potentization**.

Defence Mechanism: The ability of a living organism to resist illness and maintain health. This includes, but is more than, the immune system.

Expectoration: The coughing up of mucus.

Flatulence: Gases in the digestive system.

General Symptoms: Symptoms of the whole person. When explaining them a patient will say, for example 'I ache all over', rather than 'My legs ache'. Aching all over is a general symptom and is more important in choosing the homeopathic remedy. A symptom of the legs or any one part of the body is a *particular* **symptom**.

Immune System: The system in the body that fights infection.

Law of Cure: A medical law formulated by Dr Constantine Hering in the 19th century. Briefly, it states that healing begins within the patient and works its way outwards.

Law of Similarity: This states that a substance that can cause a certain set of symptoms in a healthy person can, when given in the appropriate way, cure that set of symptoms in a sick person.

Materia Medica: This Latin term is used to refer to the **symptom picture** of a remedy and to the books that describe the symptom pictures of homeopathic remedies.

Modality: Anything that makes a symptom, or the whole patient, better or worse.

117

Mucus Membranes: The 'inner skin' or linings of the body, such as the surfaces of the lungs and digestive system.

Orifices: The openings of the body, e.g., mouth, anus, etc.

Orthodox Medicine: *See* **Allopathic Medicine** and **Conventional Medicine**.

Placebo: A treatment that contains no medicine, for example, unmedicated pills.

Polychrest: A term used in homeopathy to describe a remedy that may be needed for many different kinds of illness.

Potency: The potency of a homeopathic remedy is the number of times it has been potentized (*see* below).

Potentization: The process of preparing a homeopathic medicine by repeated methodical dilution and shaking.

Proving: The testing of homeopathic medicines on human volunteers.

Relapse: Getting worse again after getting better.

Remedy: The term used most often to refer to a homeopathic medicine.

Remedy Picture: The result of the **proving** of a homeopathic remedy. The remedy picture includes all the symptoms that a remedy can cause and cure – far more symptoms than any one patient will ever have. The remedy picture (or symptom picture) also conveys the character and the themes of the remedy, which are patterns in the symptoms. These make the remedy pictures much easier to understand and remember.

Repertory: A book or part of a book that is an index of symptoms. After each symptom is a list of all the remedies that may cure that symptom. By cross-referencing, the one remedy that covers the whole **symptom picture** can be found. This cross-referencing is called *repertorisation*.

Rubric: A symptom listed in a repertory.

Sac lac: Milk sugar, the usual substance used as the base for homeopathic tablets.

Similarity: *See* Law of Similarity.

Similimum: The Latin term for the similar remedy, i.e., the correct homeopathic remedy.

Succussion: The shaking process used in **potentization**.

Suppression: The control, or driving inwards, of symptoms or illnesses.

Susceptibility: Vulnerability, or openness to, illness or things that can cause illness. This is caused by a flawed defence mechanism in the patient.

Symptom: Any disturbance of healthy functioning. Symptoms can be classified in many ways e.g., whether they are **general** or particular, by their severity and according to disease categories.

Symptom Picture: All the important symptoms of a patient (or of a remedy) stated in such a way as to convey the nature of the patient (or remedy).

Tinctures: Unpotentized medicines in liquid form. They are used as the starting point for **potentization**, or sometimes diluted 5 drops per tablespoon to make a lotion for external applications (e.g. *calendula*).

Vital Energy: The energy of living things that maintains life and health, and heals wounds and disease. Homeopathic remedies stimulate the vital energy.

REMEDY ABBREVIATIONS

Abbreviation	Latin name	Common name
Acon.	Aconitum Napellus	Aconite
All. cep.	Allium Cepa	Red Onion
Ant. tart.	Antimonium Tartaricum	Tartar Emetic
Apis (apis mel.)	Apis Mellifica	Honey Bee
Arn.	Arnica Montana	The Fall Herb
Ars. (ars. alb.)	Arsenicum Album	White Arsenic
Bell.	Belladonna	Deadly Nightshade
Bellis	Bellis Perennis	Daisy
Bry.	Bryonia	White Bryony
Cal.	Calendula Officinalis	Small Marigold
Canth.	Cantharis	Spanish Fly
Carbo veg.	Carbo Vegetabilis	Wood Charcoal
Caust.	Causticum	Caustic Potash
Cham.	Chamomilla Matricaria	German Chamomile
Cina.	Cina Officinalis	Wormseed
Coff.	Coffea Tosta	Roasted Coffee
Coloc.	Colocynthis	Bitter Cucumber
Dros.	Drosera Rotundifolia	Sundew
Eup. perf.	Eupatorium Perfoliatum	Boneset
Euphr.	Euphrasia	Eyebright
Ferr. phos.	Ferrum Phosphoricum	Iron Phosphate
Gels.	Gelsemium Sempervirens	Yellow Jasmine
Ham.	Hamamelis	Witch Hazel
Hep. (Hep. Sulph.)	Hepar Sulphuris Calcareum	Calcium Sulphide
Hyp.	Hypericum Perfoliatum	St John's Wort
Ign.	Ignatia Amara	St Ignatius' Bean
Ipec.	Ipecacuanha	——
Kali Bich.	Kali Bichromicum	Potassium Bichromate

REMEDY ABBREVIATIONS

Abbreviation	Latin name	Common name
Kali Carb.	Kali Carbonicum	Potassium Carbonate
Lach.	Lachesis	Venom of Bushmaster Snake
Led.	Ledum Palustre	Marsh Tea
Lyc.	Lycopodium Clavatum	Club Moss
Mag. Phos.	Magnesia Phosphorica	Magnesium Phosphate
Merc. (Merc. Sol.)	Mercurius Solubilis	Mercury (Quicksilver)
Nat. Mur.	Natrum Muriaticum	Common Salt
Nux Vom.	Nux Vomica	Poison Nut
Op.	Opium	Juice of White Poppy
Petr.	Petroleum	Crude Oil
Phos.	Phosphorus	White Phosphorus
Podo.	Podophyllum	May Apple
Puls.	Pulsatilla Nigricans	Wind Flower (Pasque Flower)
Rad. Brom.	Radium Bromide	——
Rheum	Rheum	Eastern Rhubarb
Rhus Tox.	Rhus Toxicodendron	Poison Ivy
Rumex.	Rumex Crispus	Yellow Dock
Ruta.	Ruta Graveolens	Common Rue
Sars.	Sarsaparilla	Wild Liquorice
Sep.	Sepia	Ink of the Cuttlefish
Sil.	Silica	Flint (Rock Crystal)
Spong.	Spongia Tosta	Roasted Sponge
Sulph.	Sulphur	Flowers of Sulphur
Staph.	Staphysagria	Stavesacre
Symph.	Symphytum	Comfrey
Tabac.	Tabacum	Tobacco
Urt. (Urt Urens)	Urtica Urens	Dwarf Stinging Nettle

FURTHER READING

Homeopathy: Medicine of the New Man by George Vithoulkas (Thorsons, England, 1985). An inspiring read by one of the world's leading homeopaths.

INTRODUCTORY BOOKS

The Complete Homeopathy Handbook by Miranda Castro (Macmillan, England, 1990). Similar to *New Perspectives: Homeopathy* in its subject matter, but larger and more comprehensive.

The Complete Family Guide by Dr Christopher Hammond (Element Books, 1995). An illustrated introductory book.

ADVANCED BOOKS

The Science of Homeopathy by George Vithoulkas (Thorsons, England, 1986). An essential textbook.

Homeopathy as Art And Science by Dr Elizabeth Wright Hubbard (Beaconsfield Publishers). This selection of writings includes *A Brief Study Course in Homeopathy*, which is excellent.

Homeopathic Drug Pictures by Margaret Tyler (Health Science Press, England, 1970). A lively and thorough *materia medica* of over 100 homeopathic remedies.

Materia Medica of Homeopathic Medicines by S R Phatak (Indian Books and Periodicals Syndicae). A good reference book used by many homeopaths on a daily basis.

Repertory of the Homeopathic Materia Medica by James Tyler Kent. This repertory, or one of the modern versions that include important additional material, is essential for a serious student.

Emotional Healing with Homeopathy by Peter Chappell (Element Books, 1993). This book explains self-help for emotional problems and connects homeopathy with psychotherapy.

Useful Addresses

AFRICA
African Homeopathic
Medical Foundation
PO Box 131
Nempi
Oru LGA
Imo State
Nigeria

Homeopathic Society
of South Africa
PO Box 9658
Johannesburg 2000
South Africa

W Last Pharmacy
PO Box 407
Johannesburg 2000
South Africa

AUSTRALIA
Australian
Association of
Professional
Homeopaths
PO Box 4052
Daisy Hill 4127
Queensland

The Australian
Federation of
Homeopaths
PO Box 806
Spit Junction
NSW 2088

Australian Institute
of Homeopathy
21 Bulah Close
Berdwra Heights
NSW 2082

Brauer Biotherapies
(Pharmacy)
1 Para Road
Tanunda
S. Australia 5352

Martin and Pleasance
PO Box 4
Collingwood
Victoria 3066
Australia

Society of Classical
Homeopaths
2nd Floor
Paxton House
90 Pilt Street
Sydney 2000

CANADA
Canadian Society of
Homeopaths
87 Meadowland
Drive West
Nepean,
Ontario K2G2R9

Vancouver Centre for
Homeopathy
2246 Spruce Street
Vancouver
BC V6H 2P3

FRANCE
Societé Medical de
Biotherapie
62 rue Beaubourg
75003 Paris

Centre d'Etudes
Homoeopathiques de
France
228 Boulevard
Raspail
75014 Paris

IRELAND
The Irish Society of
Homeopaths
32 Strand Street
Cloghae Head
Co. Louth

NEW ZEALAND
Institute of Classical
Homeopathy
24 West Haven Drive
Tawa, Wellington

Len Hooper
Pharmacy
104 Oxford Terrace
Epuni
Lower Hutt

The New Zealand
Homeopathic Society
PO Box 67-095
Mount Eden
Auckland 3

UK
Ainsworths's
Homoeopathic
Pharmacy
38 New Cavendish
Street
London W1M 7LH

British Homeopathic
Association
27a Devonshire
Street
London
W1N 1RJ

Buxton and Grant
176 Whiteladies
Road,
Bristol BS8 2XU

College of
Homeopathy
26, Clarendon Rise
London SE13 6JR

Freeman's
Pharmaceutical and
Homeopathic
Chemists
7 Eaglesham Road
Clarkston, Glasgow

Galen
Homoeopathics
Lewell Mill
West Stafford
Dorchester
Dorset
DT2 8AN

The Hahnemann
Society
Humana Education
Centre
Avenue Lodge
Bounds Green Road
London N22 4EU

Helios Homeopathic
Pharmacy
92 Camden Road
Tunbridge Wells
Kent TN1 2QP

The Homeopathic
Supply Co.
Fairview
4 Nelson Road
Sheringham
Norfolk NR26 8BU

London College of
Classical
Homeopathy
Morley College
61 Westminster
Bridge Road
London SE1 7HG

Glasgow
Homoeopathic
Hospital
1000 Great Western
Road
Glasgow G12

Midlands College of
Homoeopathy
186 Wolverhampton
Street
Dudley
West Midlands
DY1 3AD

A. Nelson & Co. Ltd.
73, Duke Strreet
London
W1M 6BY

Northern College of
Homeopathic
Medicine
Swinburn House
Swinburn Street
Gateshead NE8 1AX

The Royal London
Homoeopathic
Hospital
Great Ormond Street
London WC1N 3HR

The Small School of
Homoeopathy
Out of the Blue Lane
North Street,
Cromford
Derbyshire DE4 3RG

The Society of
Homoeopaths
2 Artisan Road
Northampton
NN1 4HU

Weleda (UK) Ltd.
Heanor Road
Ilkeston
Derbyshire
DE7 8DR

USA
American
Association of
Homoepathic
Pharmacies
PO Box 2273
Falls Church
Virginia, VA 22042

American
Foundation for
Homeopathy
1508 S. Garfield
Alhambra, CA 91801

American Institute of
Homeopathy
1585 Glencoe St
Ste 44
Denver
CO 80220-1338

Boericke and Tafel
Inc.
1011 Arch Street
Philadelphia
PA 19107
and
2381-T Circadian
Way
Santa Rosa
CA 95407

Boiron-Bornemann
6 Campus Blvd
Newtown Square
PA 19073

Dolisos
3014 Rigel Ave
Las Vegas
NV 89102

Foundation for
Homeopathic
Education and
Research
5916 Chabot Crest
Oakland, CA 94618

Foundation for
Homeopathic
Education and
Research
2124 Kittredge Street
Berkeley, CA 94704

Hahnemann Medical
Clinic
1918 Bonita Street
Berkeley, CA 94704

Homeopathic
Council for Research
and Education
50 Park Avenue
New York, NY 10016

Homeopathic
Medical Society of
New Mexico
122 Dartmouth
Albuquerque
NM 87106

Homeopathic
Medical Society of
Pennsylvania
Henshaw Health
Center
10 Skyport Road
Mechanicsburg
PA 17055

The Homeopathic
Pharmacopeia
Convention of the
United States
1500 Massachusetts
Avenue NW
Washington
DC 20005

International
Foundation for
Homeopathy
2366 Eastlake
Avenue E, Ste 301
Seattle, WA 98102

John Bastyr College
of Naturopathic
Medicine
1408 NE 45th St
Seattle, WA 98105

Longevity Pure
Medicines
9595 Wiltshire Blvd
*502
Beverley Hills
CA 90212

Luyties
Pharmaceutical Co
4200-T Laclede
Avenue
St Louis, MO
6318-2815

National Center for
Homeopathy
801 North Fairfax St,
Ste 306
Alexandria, VA
22314

New York
Homeopathic
Medical Society
110-56 71st Avenue,
Ste 1-H
Forest Hills, NY
113751

Ohio State
Homeopathic
Medical Society
800 Compton Road,
Ste 24
Cincinnati, OH
45231

Southern
Homeopathic
Medical Association
10418 Whitehead
Street
Fairfax, VA 22030

Standard
Homeopathic Co
204 T W 131st St
Los Angeles, CA
90061-1618

Washington
Homeopathic
Products
124 Fairfax St
Berkeley Springs
WV 25411

INDEX